Career Planning:

A Nurse's Guide To Career Advancement

Patricia Winstead-Fry, PhD, RN
University of Vermont
School of Nursing

Pub. No. 41-2295

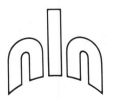

National League for Nursing • New York

ISBN 0-88737-462-X

Manufactured in the United States of America

Contents

Introduction

This book, like many things in life, has gone through several alterations in the course of development. Throughout, the most exciting part of writing this book has been the career stories shared with me by the nurses. Their careers all began at different points over a 30-year period; their paths have been varied and so reflect the experiences of women in a changing world.

The nurses who answered questions about their career development were selected because they were identified as being successful in novel/complex practice either by the nursing executive in a practice setting or by the dean of their nursing school. I sought "winners" and asked them how they planned their careers. (A copy of the questionnaire is included in Appendix A.) All of the nurses had at least a baccalaureate degree in nursing.

I wrote this book on career development for two reasons: First, because the prevailing career-development literature appears too hierarchical; that is, it assumes that one graduates from college and moves through a series of steps, usually ever higher, until some maximum level of success is achieved. Such literature is not very sensitive to women and child bearing/rearing issues. It is also limited in understanding women in a predominately female profession. Such literature is likewise insensitive to persons who may move laterally in their careers. I think lateral movement is important in looking at nursing because there are expert practitioners who may not want to move into management. In much of the career-development literature, such persons would either be considered failures or they could not be accounted for.

Secondly, today's nursing career opportunities are so diversified: There is an impressive number of "winners" who are employed in settings unheard of several years ago. Even more impressive is to think that I specifically asked the deans and nurse executives who nominated the participating nurses *not* to select entrepreneurs, as the National League for Nursing's book, *Entrepreneuring: A Nurse's Guide to Starting a Business*, covers this phenomenon quite well.

This book makes no claim to be a qualitative study of the state of nursing today. It is more in the tradition of Sheehey's *Passages*, that is, it is a discussion of important issues and events that shape the lives of nurses who are successful.

Each chapter begins with quotes from successful nurses. These are followed by comments, a self-assessment exercise, and in a few chapters, what I label "loose ends": ideas, sometimes free associations, evoked by the nurse's comments or the literature. They are not well developed in my mind or in the literature, but I thought someone might find them useful.

Finally, a note to the successful nurse participants: I tried to include each of you at least once. At times your handwriting left me baffled. If I changed a word, it was probably because I misread it. I also took the editorial prerogative of correcting punctuation. I promised you anonymity if you requested it. There were two of you who checked the space that allowed me to identify you, but then crossed your name off the questionnaire. Two others marked both the spaces, thus saying that I could identify you and simultaneously saying that I couldn't. In all of these instances, I protected anonymity. I decided that if I were to err, it would be in the direction of caution. I am very grateful for the time you spent with that lengthy questionnaire, and didn't think you would mind if I corrected spelling and punctuation. I wish I could have a party and meet each of you! What a great group!

PAT WINSTEAD-FRY, PHD, RN

To the successful nurses who answered my questionnaire
and
to successful nurses everywhere

PART ONE

The Process of
Career Planning

Career Selection

CHARACTERISTICS OF A CAREER

Most available career-planning/development literature distinguishes a career from a job. The characteristics of a career generally include choice, personal satisfaction, some degree of security, opportunity for continual growth, meaningful responsibility, and personal rewards. All of these themes, plus some other themes from nursing's historically feminist past recur in the comments of successful nurses that follow.

The nurse historian, Dr. Ellen Baer (1982), has examined the different social ideologies that influenced nursing in its early development in her doctoral dissertation, *The Conflictive Social Ideology of American Nursing: 1893, A Microcosm.* Baer identifies and discusses five ideals, embraced in varying degrees by Florence Nightingale, Isabel Hampton Robb, and Linda Richards. At times these ideals conflict with one another and they are certainly not clearly distinct from one another. The five ideals Baer outlines are: nurses as women who are characterized by certain duties and gifts; the role of religion and morality in the "call" to be a nurse; economics and social class involved in the work of nurses; the type of education/training to prepare for nurses' work; and the type of organizational structure in which nursing education and practice takes place.

The following quotes may sound strange to us today, but they were accepted and typical in turn-of-the-century discussions of nursing:

> That, while it is not at all essential to combine religious exercises with nursing, it is believed that such a union would be eminently conducive to the welfare of the sick in all public institutions.

The nurse's work is a ministry; it should be consecrated service, performed in the spirit of Christ who made himself of no account but went about being good.

Absolute and unquestioning obedience must be the foundation of the nurse's work, and to this end complete subordination of the individual to her work as a whole is as necessary for her as for the soldier.

The first quote is from the American Medical Association's Committee on the Training of Nurses, published in 1896. The second is from Hampton Robb's *Nursing Ethics* (1893). The third is a comment made by Lavinia Dock in 1893. Themes of woman, calling, and values, especially caring, are repeated in the comments of some of the successful nurses. Interestingly, when these themes are evoked, the nurse's age is not a factor, that is, older nurses do not tend to refer to these aspects of a traditionally feminine life more so than their younger colleagues.

Not all of the successful nurses repeated feminist themes from nursing history. For many, nursing was clearly a wise business decision. Such nurses discuss being able to work any shift, anywhere in the country, as nursing's advantage as a career choice. Like any successful career person, they talk of opportunities for advancement, financial rewards, the opportunity to express important aspects of self, and the ability to foresee and capitalize on market trends. But let them comment.

STORIES OF SUCCESSFUL NURSES

I went to see the movie *Magnificent Obsession* and wanted to be an operating-room nurse. My friends laughed at me. I showed them! I always perceived nursing as a career since I believe I have choices in life and accept responsibility for my actions and decisions.

A. Uruburu

I was attracted to the nursing profession because of

- the opportunity to serve, and probably to be a bit of a martyr, which was undoubtedly an outgrowth of my Catholic grammar-school education's emphasis on serving others.

- the opportunity of working with people. I was, myself, enjoying and being enjoyed by others so I reasoned that I would do well working with the public.

- a beloved aunt, who lived with my family, was a health care worker and derived satisfaction from her work. She had dropped out of nursing school in England because of an illness. Her oldest sister, my mother, had also wanted to become a nurse, but her father would not permit her to go to England from Ireland, and she came to America instead. I have always associated nursing with my aunt, though I am sure that however much I repressed my mother's unmet goals, they did influence my decision.

- the opportunity to always be able to work day or night, seven days a week, anywhere in the country. Such concerns were uppermost in my mind because my mother was widowed when I was five and she had to raise four of us herself.

I believe I always viewed nursing as a career. As a matter of fact, one of the pulls to nursing was that I would be able to manage a family and achieve a measure of self-development and self-satisfaction in nursing without completely giving up either.

This perception was strongly influenced in my high-school education. I attended an all-female school where I was constantly reminded that I was gifted and expected to achieve. It was there that I first learned about, and was taught by, women with a PhD or EdD, and remember thinking I'd get a PhD one day. I knew I would go to college, and Hunter College was opening a nursing program. I went to see the chairperson about it and knew by my junior year in high school that I would go to Hunter. At Hunter, I was constantly reminded that I was being educated as a professional nurse and that I was expected to be in the forefront of the profession's development once I graduated. Education versus training and profession versus vocation were frequent topics for discussion.

The multiple factors for me were the array of intelligent women who had educated me beginning in kindergarten. The vast majority were admirable, strong, and fair. Some spoke of their spouses and children, and others talked of their friends and activities; all in all they did more than one thing and were marvelous role models.

E. L. Gallagher

I started college at age 50, after raising a family of eight children. My first chosen profession was homemaker. When I started school, my first desire was just to go and take some fun classes. Then I wanted to see if I could do the hard stuff. I couldn't. I flunked test after test, but I had eight children, eight in-laws, and 16 grandchildren watching. If I quit, just because it was hard, then I would be sending a message I didn't want to portray to my family that is, "If it's hard, just quit." I couldn't do that; so I stuck out the second quarter. Then I took human anatomy. With that class came a lab. One afternoon on my way home from the lab, I stopped off at my friend's office on campus and said, "Today, we got to play with real live, dead bodies." I was so excited because I had been trying to memorize the muscle attachments on paper and they just wouldn't click. When I saw the real thing, I became ecstatic. My friend said, "Go declare your major. You're making me sick. If you get that excited over dead bodies, you should be a nurse." I made an appointment with the college of nursing, found out what I had to do, and went for it! One class I had to take three times, but from the first interview, I never lost sight of the end goal.

I never saw nursing as a paycheck. The fact is that I never planned to work even after I graduated. I just thought it would be nice to have a degree. Somewhere along the way, however, I realized how very stupid that would have been. Too much sweat, hard work, stress, and tears, let alone the tuition, had gone into obtaining the degree not to use it. I also realized I would never be a nurse just by going to school. I learned to be a nurse after I graduated and worked in the hospital. I chose to do my synthesis course on a medical-surgical unit where I could get tons of experience. By the help of the Lord and through prayer and searching, I found the best preceptor for me that there was. She was the age of my children, but she was like a mother to me. She was so patient and never belittled me or chewed me out or criticized me. I was at such a low ego point in my schooling that had she done any of the above, I feel as though it would have been the end of me. It would have validated my feelings of inability and worthlessness. It was because of her that I quit my part-time job at another hospital and went to work full-time at Holy Cross Hospital after graduation. During the clinical courses of school, I realized how much I loved being a nurse. To serve anyone always feeds the server. To me, nursing is the opportunity to serve, and to get a paycheck on top of that is icing on the cake.

B. Frampton

Cornball though it sounds, I wanted to be a nurse because I like people and I thought it would be personally rewarding and very interesting. I believed I would be a happier, satisfied human being if I could help folks in some way that they would deem helpful. I had my first experience with nurses when I was eight or nine and had a tonsilectomy and adenoidectomy. My grandmother's good friend was the director of nursing at the small community hospital where I was a patient. I remember thinking how wonderful the student nurses were who took care of me and who comforted me. I thought nursing was something I should consider doing when I grew up.

I believe I always viewed nursing as a career. I can't remember ever thinking of nursing as just a job with a paycheck. I made it my business to find out as much as I could about nursing before making the decision to go to nursing school. I spent the summer between my sophomore and junior years in high school as a pre-nursing aide at a large city hospital. I lived in the nurses' home, attended classes, and worked in the hospital. I spent lots of time on and off duty asking the student nurses questions. I asked the registered nurses more questions and I kept my eyes opened. Once accepted at a diploma school, I did have a mentor, a wonderful person and a great teacher. We are friends to this day, though she is retired now.

I did experience a critical incident—an unexpected divorce. I had been out of nursing raising a family for about 11 years. I had to decide whether to return to nursing or to change careers. I gave this lots of thought. I had been happy with my earlier career choice, so I decided to stay in nursing. I knew nursing had changed. I consulted with my first mentor and soon realized that I could not expect to advance without at least an undergraduate degree. I also consulted an old friend. She was an instructor at the University of Maryland. She put me in touch with the RN-to-BSN program. I had to start from ground zero. I took 60 credits at my community college, challenged for about 28 credits, and finally got into Maryland. I went full-time for one year and received the BS in nursing.

Somewhere along the line, while at the community college, I knew I would not be able to pursue one career goal unless I had a master's degree. Since I was "in the groove" and was doing well as an adult student, I stayed on for the master's program in psychiatric nursing.

The whole process of community college, the BS program and the master's program took me five years. I called it my five-year plan and let *nothing* deter me from achieving it. I later learned that I was (am) a functional, as well as a chronological oldest; so it is no surprise that nothing could deter me.

Nursing was one of the few fields available. I was encouraged by my mother to prepare for being a wife and mother. At first nursing was a job, even when it wasn't. When I had to work to support my family (my husband was in a career change) and had small children, I resented it because I wanted to be at home and "do my own thing." When I went to graduate school, it was to prove to myself (and others) that I could do it. I was incredibly successful as a graduate student and developed self-confidence. I began to see myself as a career woman—and I love it!

My first attraction to the nursing profession occurred during my high school years. However, due to a dominating grandmother, I was not allowed to pursue a career in nursing. She believed that nurses were "hand maidens" and that it was not a valuable career choice. As a result, I was shipped off to accounting school. During my childhood, I was reared to respect my elders, and therefore, did not resist my grandmother's intervention. I received an AS in accounting. Later in my life I chose to go back to school and to become a nurse. At this point, my grandmother was in a nursing home. I told her of my choice, and she still was not pleased. As my nursing education progressed, my grandmother's mental and physical condition began to deteriorate. I observed this and committed myself to "making a difference." Hence, my BSN and then my MSN as a gerontological nurse practitioner.

The career choice which I have made was a conscious and deliberate one. Because of my commitment to the elderly, I began to investigate the societal need for my choice and my career potential. This occurred during the late 1970s and early 1980s. I foresaw the "graying of America" and chose geriatrics as the field in which I could become an expert and also the place in which I could advance quickly. In five years, I predict that I will have my primary job as a gerontological nurse practitioner, continue to work collaboratively with a physician, and also maintain a private practice and a consulting business.

A. Clayman

I became a nurse solely as a means to an end. I wanted to practice nurse midwifery. I do view nursing, now that I have experience with the profession, as the most flexible profession in terms of practicing and contributing to one's area of interest.

I always viewed nursing as a career. I knew that certified nurse midwives were well-prepared, independent practitioners with great responsibility and commitment. My father was a university professor. I guess I want what I do from life because he convinced me I should and could have it all.

M. Scoville

I was first attracted to the nursing profession when I was approximately three years old and my first sibling was born. At that time, we made regular trips to the pediatrician, and I was very taken with the office nurse who was a very kind and pleasant person. I particularly liked the fact that she was dressed in white shoes, white stockings, and a very smart looking white dress. I decided that it looked very nice and that I would like to look like her someday.

Nancy Valentine

It was an arbitrary decision. I wanted to go to Canada when I was 17. My father wouldn't let me go unless I had a job or college to come back to. I applied to nursing school, took the exams, was accepted, and left for Canada. When I returned nine months later, I entered nursing school.

I began to work as an orderly in an acute-care, psychiatric setting. I was happy and challenged by the scope and perspective of this job. I observed the registered nurses and began to see that I might find fulfillment in that role. Other individuals in the work setting encouraged me to pursue this objective. I enjoyed the intensity and richness of human interrelationships in this role and found that it brought out the best in my talents. I found that this career situation excited me. My previous training and education was in philosophy, which I had studied in the university for many years. Nursing offered me an avenue in which to apply many of my analytic skills. From the beginning, I also realized that I valued women highly as peers, and that working with women brought out my maleness in a different way. This state of affairs allowed me to get in touch with who I am—a loving, caring, masculine human being who seeks meaningful interrelationships with others.

I always viewed nursing as a career of meaning and personal commitment. I came to this awareness at a very early age. Indeed I do *not* believe I ever placed great value on issues of economic security. This has lasted until, and including, the present, through my marriage of 18 years, and the births of my 2 daughters.

A desire to be with people in their pain and problems in order to relieve them, help them cope, and find ways to health. There was probably a "lady bountiful" piece in the early days, but I've come to see the art of nursing involved much more with empowerment.

I've always felt that nursing was an art and a way to share with people on an intimate and privileged level. Somehow "career/job" doesn't define my perception of what I'm about as much as the word "profession." Those who have influenced me most are some of the early religious reformers who answered the cry of the poor, Lillian Wald, and those who began the Visiting Nurse Service. Current nurses and other health care providers who see the whole person and struggle with them to prevent illness and to promote health influence me.

D. Calvani

I was looking for a major in college. My dormitory suitemate was quitting nursing and told me and her roommate all about her clinical training. She hated it! The roommate and I were intrigued and applied to the program. We are now nurses and our suitemate is very happy in her career in journalism.

When I started nursing school, I thought of nursing as a job with an added benefit of mobility and secure employment. The primary concern of my parents, who had been poor as children, during World War II in Japan and in the Depression in America, was that I go to college so I could get a good job. This influenced what I considered as possibilities and choices for majors in college. I was socialized in schools and by journals I read, and by nurses I met, to view nursing as a career.

K. Allman

I was drawn to nursing by a desire to be in the medical field and to deal directly with people in a *direct* manner, as opposed to the physician who doesn't spend a great deal of time with people. I also wanted to be able to care for others.

I have always perceived nursing as a career, which is why I chose to go to college for a degree in nursing versus attending a diploma program. Nursing is a part of my life, and my life as a nurse has a direct and immediate bearing and influence on the lives of the people (patients) I meet every day. My knowledge, experience, and skill make me a very influential person to colleagues as well as to patients. To have the responsibility that all this entails makes me a professional with a career that doesn't end after eight hours. I am responsible for lives. If I thought of nursing as a job only, then I shouldn't be a nurse. Nor should anyone else!

D. Boyle

I know from several years of personal counseling and developing self-awareness that I tend to be drawn toward the "helping" role not only professionally, but personally as well. Being the middle child in a family in conflict, I became good at mediating and smoothing over problems, and thus, was always helping others with their problems. I was also quite bright and good in science in school. Actually, my initial intent was to become a doctor, and in fact I did enroll in pre-med courses my freshman year. However, I could only obtain B's in organic chemistry and felt overwhelmed by the intense competition. I therefore chose to study nursing as an alternative, but had several years of adjusting to this decision. I struggled with a sense of second best and a covert resentment probably until two and one-half years into my practice as a registered nurse. When I began to change my perceptions of nursing and more clearly understand the special important differences between nursing and medicine, I also dealt with the issues of resentment and inferiority and how they showed up in other parts of my life.

The first two and one-half years of my practice were in an intensive care unit and in a labor and delivery suite in two different hospitals in Rhode Island. Despite being prepared for a career in nursing school, these were jobs. The professional status of nursing in 1978–80 in Rhode Island was incredibly poor. Staffing was dismal; administrative support absent; continuing education was minimal; responsibility was high, but autonomy and authority to make decisions was absent. Nurses punched time clocks and were docked pay if 15 minutes late. The charge nurse ran the show. The union rewarded longevity, not education. It was truly a "worker" mentality. Practice was not based on research, but on habit. I was clearly disenchanted with nursing.

I decided that if I was to remain in nursing, I needed to work in a more rewarding environment, and so moved to Boston to Beth Israel Hospital. I was truly amazed at the difference. Nursing identity was so clearly defined! There was a unified professional practice model in place. Over the next year or so, I actually discovered what was great about being a nurse and it became a career. After being exposed to the clinical specialist role, I wanted to go to graduate school. My head nurse supported this. She let me set my own schedule and work part-time during school. Graduate school was also extremely important in defining nursing for me, especially working with nursing diagnosis and the scope and domain of nursing concerns. The research role was exciting. The way I viewed nursing and myself have changed and I feel more empowered as well.

I was guided, I believe, to be a nurse. I remember as a senior in high school I was an accomplished pianist and planned to apply to music schools. I was filling out college applications, had written "music" in the space provided for my selected major, and found myself crossing out music and writing in nursing. I honestly cannot explain why! I enjoyed helping people (not always from a healthy, motive-free place) and was/am a compassionate and loving person. I loved biology in high school, which turned me in the direction of medicine and nursing, but all in all, I feel I was guided and not necessarily attracted to the nursing profession. When I was a young girl, I could never imagine being a nurse, so imagine my surprise when I chose to become a nurse!

I saw my few years as a nurses' aide as a job, but once I became a nurse, I truly saw it as a life-long profession. I felt I had chosen something that gave me great meaning and purpose. Something I felt was a service to humanity that also gave me the reward of much goodness. My work in the profession was as a nurse practitioner and although this expanded role gave me a sense of responsibility and meaning, I left the profession after three years of work. At this time I had my master's degree, but had lost heart in the western/allopathic way. I began to explore nutrition, herbs, and other modalities for healing. Although I kept my nursing license current, I began to explore many other alternative ways of healing.

There was a period of nine years before I returned to nursing. During that time, I did not think of myself as a nurse and actually felt embarrassed about being a nurse. I did many different jobs, none with a great deal of meaning. I was politically active around issues of women's health, disability rights, and environmental/hunger issues. These were years of self-development and explorations of who I was and what was important to me.

Six years ago, I attended a weekend for nurses in transition, many of whom were following nontraditional paths. I felt like I had come home! There were 45 nurses who shared a common vision and the woman who facilitated the weekend became a mentor for me. We have since worked together on projects and have bonded as friends. I became introduced to the American Holistic Nurses' Association, where I found another mentor and began my path of rooting in my current directions.

V. Andrus

I think my attraction to nursing began with a desire to understand how living things ticked—kind of like wanting to know more about the mystery of life. As a young teenager, I was going to be a scientist. I remember having surgery when I was about 12 and perhaps my experiences with nurses influenced my decision, although I do not remember any person talking to me or encouraging me to go into nursing. I do not remember the actual decision to become a nurse, but by the age of 14 I was telling my family that I was going to nursing school. I remember being very sure about it and never changed my goal or doubted my decision. I did not even consider a university at this time. Hospital training was all I knew about and my parents were not in a position to advise me differently.

I thought nursing was important. I knew I would be a good nurse and I wanted to be a success. I wanted my family to be proud of me and I wanted to be proud of myself.

I do not believe I ever viewed nursing as a job. However, I think I perceived early in my career that the system (hospital) perceived nursing as a job. It was clear to me that it was more important to have the job done than how the job was done. I worked for six years as a diploma nurse before returning to school for my baccalaureate.

I remember being very frustrated and angry with nursing and I seriously considered leaving, but I really loved nursing. I thought the only way to change things was to return to school. What was I frustrated with back then? I was frustrated with colleagues who I think did view nursing as a job. I was frustrated with myself for trying to do my best in a system that did not care if I did or did not. And I was frustrated by the way we treated human beings. I remember comments from senior nurses like, "It's two o'clock; time to turn the veggies." I believed back then that it didn't matter what kind of job I did because I would be advanced like everyone else—on seniority, not performance.

I always felt like I was banging my head against a brick wall because I could never do enough to feel satisfied with what I was doing. I always felt I should have done more, but no—that's not it. I always felt I should have done things differently, but I could not at that time have told you what I meant.

I did not have mentors when I was a diploma nurse, but I always had supervisors who reinforced what I believed in and who encouraged me in evaluations. The patients affirmed me more than anything. I moved quickly to achieve technical expertise. I remember thinking nursing would be better in ICU, and it was. I at least had the time to do what I believed I should be doing. I was respected and I did my work well, but there was still something missing. I did not know what, but I was not satisfied.

Returning for my BScN radically changed my beliefs about nursing. That was when I first began to view nursing as a profession, or at least a potential profession. I was mentored in school and have had mentors in school and practice since. I believe the mentors I have had and now have are critical to my professional survival. My present mentor affirms me and facilitates my struggle to go on at a time when I feel vulnerable and uncertain about where nursing is going to end up as a profession.

It was not until I received my master's degree and assumed my present position as a clinical nurse specialist that I felt like a professional nurse. I function as an autonomous practitioner with little direction from my superior. In the past two to three years I have also defined what my practice is all about. I guide my practice with a nursing theory which I believe clarifies my contribution as a nurse and guides the way I am with individuals. The theory supports my personal and professional values and beliefs. My goals in practice are now legitimized and validated in a way they have never been. I now feel great about what I do as a nurse.

G. Mitchell

I'm not sure what attracted me to nursing—probably altruism. I read something in the fifth grade about Florence Nightingale and a *Reader's Digest* condensed book about the ship H.O.P.E. They must have really inspired me because I've always thought of nursing as a vocation.

I viewed nursing as a career since I was a junior in high school when I made a choice between a diploma school and a college. It was difficult as I had a father who thought "an RN is an RN. Why spend all that money when you are going to get married and have children anyway?" After I chose the BSN route, I think I had to in my own way, demonstrate to my father that I did have a *career* in nursing.

I remember also the criticism I received for changing jobs after two or three years for better opportunities. The opportunities I was choosing early in my career involved less pay, but more autonomy, and a better life-style. I had worked from the time I was 15 in either a hospital or a nursing home as an aide. At 21, I'd already had plenty of weekend and holiday shifts, so I opted for a job in community health; after 13 months as an ICU nurse.

A divorce did prompt me into a master's program. It was education or adventure! I'd all but signed the papers to go to Brazil with the Peace Corps for three years to teach pediatric nursing. An advertisement for an outreach program from a major university attracted my interest and then the hardcore professional socialization occurred.

Cynthia Beel Bates

As long as I can remember, I wanted to be a nurse. The person who influenced me the most in that decision was an aunt who was a religious in charge of a home for unwed mothers. I would often visit her on Sundays. She was such a loving, dedicated person that I was sure nursing was what I wanted to do. My mother nearly died shortly after the birth of my youngest sister, and I remember my aunt being there at her bedside, comforting her and us. Nursing was not a job for her! It was her life and I believe that I have always felt the same about my own profession. I have volunteered for ambulance work, taught EMT courses, and usually visited the sick or elderly in my neighborhood; anyone could call me at home. It was just part of my life as a nurse.

I am the second child, the oldest girl, in a family from a small, factory town. My father was a very capable man who was never able to get a college education. The frustration he felt spurred us to go to college, even if it meant we had to find the money ourselves. Dad really encouraged us to get knowledge to improve ourselves. It was because of his encouragement that five of his children are college graduates and four have master's degrees. My mother has always been the silent supporter and the haven when times got hard. She helped us fill in financial aid forms, get jobs, and survive the pressures of getting through college. They are both still very supportive of us and are extremely proud of our accomplishments.

When it was time for me to choose a nursing school, my aunt encouraged me to choose a baccalaureate program. She had taken some college courses at St. Anselm College and saw the value of the BSN degree. I applied and was accepted at St. Anselm and began the journey toward my life-long dream. My years at St. Anselm were the beginning of my maturing process. The nursing department's philosophy instilled in us the vision that nursing is a profession and the BSN graduate must be an example of what nursing *should* be. I was often involved in a variety of activities at school and the leadership I demonstrated earned me the honor of being chosen for *Who's Who In American Colleges and Universities.*

Like many other new graduates, the first year of nursing practice was difficult. There were seven new graduates that started at Portsmouth Hospital (New Hampshire) with me, and although I was the only BSN there was a great deal of comraderie and mutual support. However, eight months after being hired, I was asked to take charge of a floor for two weeks. The director of nursing knew I was still learning, but she felt I could do the job. When someone places that much faith in you, you naturally put forth your best. I was surprised at how easy it was for me to be in charge—the leadership mode fit me well. There was also satisfaction in working independently and this led me to my second job as a visiting nurse. Because of the people skills I learned from my father and the tact I learned from mom, I did well in that job. A very difficult pregnancy cut that career short. It might have been okay just to have one baby, but I got pregnant four months after the birth of my premature son, and so I decided to stay home and take care of the family. (Family planning was not my strength!)

When the urge to return to nursing had me looking for another opportunity, the school next door to our home was looking for a nurse who could teach. I had both qualifications because I had done a fair bit of teaching; so I was a school nurse for two years. The challenge was to develop a health curriculum and keep these youngsters under control. This was not what I saw as my niche in life.

In 1978, scholarships for graduate education in nursing were readily available, so I applied to Catholic University. We sold our home in New Hampshire and moved to Bethesda, Maryland. I worked at Georgetown University Hospital while a student and enjoyed the excitement of a large, teaching hospital. School was a little challenging with a two- and a three-year-old, but learning has always been my passion and so the two years went by quickly. My husband Terry was a wonderful support in helping with the children, as well as with the writing of my thesis. My French background sometimes made my sentences a little reversed and Terry would correct my work with all of the patience of Job. I was the student representative on the curriculum development committee and again enjoyed the involvement of school activities. I was pleased to be chosen as a member of Sigma Theta Tau.

We contemplated returning to New Hampshire after receiving my degree, but we really couldn't afford to move; so I decided to look around for a job in Washington, DC. I was thrilled to be chosen for a position as clinical instructor at Sibley Memorial Hospital, especially when there had been 22 applicants. This was the beginning of my professional penchant for education. My year as an instructor was challenging and I suppose one of my strengths is that I am always changing things that do not work well. Innovation and change are always part of my life. After only one year as an instructor, I was asked to become the director of education. There were 12 instructors in my department (for 350 beds) and the administration strongly supported education. I was the spoiled kid on the block! I had the money and resources available to make some real advances in nursing practice and I jumped at the opportunity. We implemented competency-based orientation when it was still just an idea. Our year-long internship for new graduates made us the most sought-after hospital in DC. In 1982, when other hospitals were experiencing a shortage of nurses, we were turning them away. It was a real blessing to be a person with ideas and the resources to make these ideas a reality.

One would have thought that this experience would have kept me content, but I'm afraid I was looking for yet another type of challenge. Terry and I often talked about doing volunteer work in a developing country. Encouraged by a minister who had just returned from Singapore, we looked for an organization that would sponsor a family. We found what we were looking for in the Los Angeles Lay Mission Helpers. The time came for the Quinns to pack up again and head west to Los Angeles where we would have a nine-month training period before being sent overseas. St. Vincent Medical Center was looking for an instructor and was excited about the fact that I could help them develop a competency-based orientation program. The year was a rewarding one, teaching the other instructor what I had learned in developing my own program and refining that knowledge. In May 1983, we drove back to New England with the few possessions we had brought to California, and prepared to go to Papua New Guinea for the next three years.

D. Quinn

Nursing seemed to be about the only option I felt I had. Being a good, Irish Catholic girl from Boston, nursing or teaching were the only acceptable choices. Secretarial work did not interest me whatsoever, nor did joining a religious order. I was very good in science in grammar school and in high school; I liked people, particularly older people. So nursing was it. I knew I had to do something with my life.

In nursing school or as a new graduate, I did not think of nursing as a career or job. It was just a reasonable way to do something with my life. Money did not enter into the scheme of things. It was in graduate school that nursing took on more of a meaning of career for me. Graduate school was one of the best experiences ever, being exposed to people who were bright, creative, and wanted to go places and do great things with nursing. I think it was also at this time that I put more of myself into nursing, knowing that I most likely wouldn't marry and have a family, having had a hysterectomy at age 25.

I fell into nursing almost by accident. In my first 21 years, I never anticipated becoming a nurse. I viewed it as a physically difficult job with little reward. I entered college intent on becoming a medical researcher. Chemistry, however, prevented progress in that direction. While attending college, I worked at a chemical corporation in the accounting and the public relations departments. I advanced to a first-line management position. I was successful but miserable. In the midst of the structure and paperwork, I developed an ulcer. I'm so thankful for that ulcer! At that time I was making decisions based on rational logic, and the ulcer was a reason to make a career change.

I knew I wanted to be in the health profession; I knew I needed people contact. I chose nursing because of job availability and security.

My first semester in nursing school, junior year, I became totally committed to the profession. Nursing became my identity. My enthusiasm was so great it was difficult for me to understand why everyone did not want to be a nurse. My first job as a staff nurse was equally enthusiastic. I was involved in creating and implementing programs such as primary nursing, preceptor programs, levels of practice, and participative management. During that time, I wrote my thoughts on nursing to *R.N.* magazine. The comments were published. *R.N.* said, I "captured the spirit of nursing."

To me, nursing is power. Through nursing, I possess the power to change the world around me. On a daily basis, I can change fear to understanding, discomfort to comfort, dependence to independence, and at times, even death to life. Actually, fear, discomfort, and dependence were primary problems that I addressed in 90 percent of my care plans. (It was a time prior to nursing diagnosis.) I just wrote what I did every day.

I was attracted to the nursing profession approximately 10 years ago because of a desire to help individuals. I saw it as an opportunity to use a wide range of knowledge, as well as the direct hands-on care with individuals experiencing debilitating or life-threatening illnesses.

I first viewed nursing as a career when I entered the expanded nursing role. Prior to that time, I saw my role as more of the 8-hour-a-day, 40-hour-a-week employee receiving a paycheck. When I became more autonomous in my opportunities as a clinical nurse specialist, I began to view it as a 24-hour-a-day career with advancement opportunity. I was now responsible for my own scheduling, my own goal setting, and outcomes which offered me a greater opportunity for satisfaction and advancement.

M. Schulte

Even though it has only been 12 years since I entered nursing school, I have difficulty recalling one particular thing that attracted me to nursing. I think probably that it is a "helping" profession. I have always been a very goal-oriented person and felt like I needed to declare a major prior to beginning school. I don't know if subconsciously I felt like nursing was a good career for a woman.

In general, I have always thought of nursing as a career. If it was just a job, I could surely find an easier way to make money. If not for the personal rewards and the feeling of doing something really important and meaningful, I perhaps would have left nursing. Because the personal rewards and the feeling of doing something meaningful are such strong motivators for me, I have never seriously considered leaving the profession. I think that I have always thought of nursing as a career because of the role models I have come in contact with. One of my instructors in school was a really sharp, intelligent, professional woman who just seemed to know everything, and handled anything that came up. I want to and hope to have influenced others as she influenced me.

C. Mulvenon

I was attracted to nursing because it seemed *practical* in terms of availability of jobs with reasonable pay. I had never worked in a hospital and had no relatives or friends in nursing. I understood very little about the profession when I chose it.

During my schooling, I viewed nursing as a career. I think this had less to do with nursing than the fact I was very much focusing on career, getting out of school in four years, and starting out on my own. I knew it was important for me to like my job. It was by luck, I think, that I liked nursing. I had no mentor and no guidance. I think as I progressed through the curriculum, I had role models among my professors and the staff nurses, and admired their intelligence and independence. I think I thought it was a glamorous profession!

J. Sheehy

Initially, I was attracted to the nursing profession because my mother is a nurse. It sparked my interest. As a result, I wanted to and did volunteer as a candy striper and did not have a positive experience. I thought of other professions, but eventually came back to nursing. I got a part-time job in the hospital and enjoyed it. What attracted me to nursing was the challenge mentally of having to be "on top" of things. I enjoyed working with people (pretty stereotyped!) and I enjoyed the intricacies of the impact of nursing on the human system. The challenge and variety of nursing opportunities *keeps* me interested in nursing.

I believe initially I saw nursing as a job, a means of support financially for me, even after my BSN. It wasn't until I was fully over the orientation of my first job that I got increasingly involved in the nursing profession. I was more open to looking at nursing as a career, either because I fell more "in love" with it or because my horizons were broadened beyond what I was in school. I guess over a period of 6 to 18 months after I graduated from the BSN program, my idea and knowledge of nursing as a career grew. During the next two years, I got more involved in professional organizations and additional professional activities. I was able to choose areas of interest to develop further, was able to take on additional responsibility, and saw more personal rewards as a result of these.

R. Brown

2

Career Planning

No, I have not done career mapping. After graduating, I decided pediatrics was where my heart was. I worked with children for two years and loved it. I then moved to Austin because my significant other was going to attend the University of Texas. I wanted to work on my master's. I was not able to get a full-time job on a pediatric unit and ended up on a general surgery floor in a large private hospital. I thought it would be temporary, but quickly knew it was a good place for me to be. I was a staff nurse for one year and then was a staff development specialist for two years. Computers quickly became my focus. I was chosen by the vice president to be the health information systems nursing representative for Seton Medical Center in the Daughters of Charity West Central Providence. This is a part-time job and I am simultaneously a charge nurse. In five years, I hope to have completed my MSN.

E. Godfrey

My career planning up to this point revolves around being a clinical specialist working directly with patients. I never formally discussed or planned how or when I would achieve my master's degree. When I was younger, I just realized that having my diploma was not enough. I wanted more from myself. It took me six years to complete my BSN, and I thought, "Why stop here? Another two years and I would have a master's." By that time, I knew that I wanted to be a clinical specialist so I could have a broader impact on patient care and on colleagues. In five years, I hope to still be working as a clinical specialist. Also, I would like to be more well known in my field. I want to publish more than I have and be involved with research.

M. Finnell

I have not done any formal career planning by a specific method other than my own personal style. I recently left an administrative position in a large department of a major medical center in New York to pursue a sales position in the private sector with a company providing home infusional therapies such as enteral therapy, TPN, and antibiotic and chemotherapy. I am not enjoying this position at all and am actively looking for a way back into oncology research. I know that I will not go back to patient care having experienced the physical and emotional fatigue others call "burn out". Interestingly, I have never missed the patient care even though I loved it at the time. This is all my way of saying that for the first time in my career, I have no five-year plan. This makes me a little apprehensive, but I know that I will find something that I will be qualified to do and that I can enjoy.

I planned on pursuing management in nursing after my children started school. Two years ago, the assistant vice president for nursing asked me to be an acting nurse manager in a 54-bed surgical unit. I had worked on this unit for seven years. I did so, remained in the position for six months, and enjoyed management. I accepted an assistant nurse manager position on the same unit. I then applied for the nurse manager position I currently hold six months later.

I entered management about five years before I thought I would. My plans for further education are to start graduate school and work on my master's in hospital management or business. I am undecided at this point. I will not start school for at least another three years because my husband is currently working on his master's degree.

I have not done career planning in any formal way. My career path was paved by an intuitive sense regarding the areas of nursing practice I wished to experience, and the need to grow and develop the skills for establishing a scientific base to my practice. These things have led me to pursue and complete a PhD program and to lay the groundwork for a research career.

I'd like to be able to say that I did something as systematic as career planning, but I'm not quite sure that it happened that way. After I finished my undergraduate degree in nursing, I expected to pursue graduate education at some point. I like being a student and value the opportunity to learn in a structured environment. However, I would not have predicted the path I followed.

My professional career has evolved from a variety of experiences. For example, right out of my baccalaureate program, I received a full scholarship to a graduate program in psychiatric nursing—the area of nursing I was most intrigued with in my undergraduate program. During my first semester in the graduate program, it became clear to me that I was not cut out for psychiatric nursing, at least not in the locked wards where they placed me for clinical experiences. On my exit interview from the graduate program, someone suggested I consider public health nursing. I followed that suggestion and found that I loved being out in the community and working with people over time. My experience as a public health nurse working in very poor neighborhoods where people had limited access to health led to my becoming a nurse practitioner. My preparation as a nurse practitioner provided an entry into the academic environment as a place to work, and so on. Each step has led to the next. Part of the progression has been intuitive, following what seemed to be the next appropriate step. Part has been guided by my own expectations/desires for education, and thus the need to enter and reenter school at various intervals.

At present, I am combining practice and research. Five years from now, I hope to have the structure for an ongoing research program in place. I am not sure whether I will be working in an academic or service institution—that part has yet to evolve.

Yes, I career planned. I identified specific goals while in my undergraduate program. I wanted an MSN to expand my role and to increase my flexibility. I planned to achieve the PhD after ten years of practice to increase my economic rewards with a growing family. In five years, I anticipate working in nursing half-time in an organization and expanding my private practice. I envision having only a half-time private practice in the next ten years.

K. Bentley

I am not quite sure what career mapping is. My career seems to have unfolded. I guess I would call my progress intuitive sense. I have been fortunate in my life to have made healthy and positive decisions for myself. The same has been true of my career. I have done in my career as I have done in my life. I saw people who were doing work that I admired, whose practice and philosophy I respected, who had a strong knowledge base and ability to share it with others and I would seek to emulate them.

My first role model in nursing was my first head nurse. She was known for her skill in management and staff development; so I interviewed with her. Her communication skills were well developed, clear, and direct. I actively sought to learn this from her and enlisted her help in my development. My next mentor was a geriatric nurse specialist. Her clinical skill and knowledge base seemed never-ending. She was also an excellent speaker and trainer. I spent as much time with her as I could. I pursued my own education form by requesting clinical consults on many elderly patients to learn from her approach. I continue to have a commitment to the dignified and individualized care of the older population. I had a natural interest in chemical restraints with the elderly and soon learned their ineffective and often harmful effects on patient's outcomes.

At this same time, I noticed that the care of our substance-abusing patients was often without direction and expertise. The same learning process could not take place for me because there was not an addictions nurse specialist to model myself after. I started an interest group for nurses interested in the addicted population and we began to educate ourselves through article sharing and reading, thoughtful discussions, and outside speakers.

One speaker in particular became and continues to be my current mentor. She suggested I attend a clinical fellow program at the Center for Addiction Studies that recently opened at her agency. In the program, I learned about addictions from the experts from a multiplicity of disciplines. I also had the opportunity to work as a drug counselor to addicted clients in a methadone maintenance clinic. It was through school that I began a supervisory relationship with Janice Kauffman, RN, that continues today. My hospital supported me two days per week to attend classes to do my required clinical work. The more I learned about the addicted population, the greater wealth of information I had to contribute to patient care at Beth Israel. The more suggestions I offered nurses for patient care, the more credibility I established. The greater my credibility, the more frequently I was called to consult on patient care on other units. It was at this point that my nurse manager offered to support me to spend one-half of my week as a nurse consultant and liaison. What I offer to nursing practice and patient care in addictions is similar to what my role model and mentor in geriatrics offered to me and my patients.

In five years, I would like to have finished my master's program in psychiatric-mental health nursing. I hope to continue as a consultant/liaison and trainer regarding issues that arise when caring for the addicted person. AIDS is another specialty of mine and together with addiction will be vitally important to patient care in the next decade. Public policy is important to me as well. Whatever it is I will be doing in five years, I know I am committed to direct patient care.

M. Gorman

Early in my career I depended on my intuitive sense of career moves.

Now that I am so successful and feel I have a great deal to lose by a "wrong" career move, I trust myself less and have consulted career specialists. I am in the process right now of mapping out my next five years. I also spend a great deal of time meditating and self-reflecting, trying to put myself where I am supposed to "be" at this time.

H. Anderson

Career planning is an integral part of success. If you don't plan, you will not know which opportunity to pursue. No wind is the right wind when you have not set a course! Basically, I have ten-year plans, five-year plans, three-year plans, and one-year-to-six-month plans. The importance is to analyze each to see if they are congruent and build upon each other. With this concept, each job is a stepping stone and a challenge. Burn-out tends to be curtailed by this optimistic course. I pursued a bachelors degree first because I wanted to teach eventually. However, before starting my masters, I worked full-time in a CCU intensive care unit. I am presently in an educator role, covering cardiopulmonary aspects of nursing. I work with the specialty units, ER, OR, RR, ICU, and stepdown units. My masters will be in cardiopulmonary nursing (MSN,R). Upon completion of my masters, I want to enter a university setting and accomplish my doctorate and publish.

J. Mueller

I have never consciously career planned. At certain critical junctures in life, choices have appeared (probably at times where I could see them). I "discovered" meditation in my life in 1983, after I completed my master's degree. I had no clear-cut idea about what type of job I wanted. But lo and behold a two-year position opened as a behavior medicine fellow which required both a master's degree and meditation experience. I got the position and spent two years learning/teaching behavioral interventions for hypertensive patients in an interdisciplinary setting. After that, I did not know what would happen, but a new position was created in a pain center. They were looking for someone with interdisciplinary experience and a behavioral medicine background. I got to create a new role for a CNS at that clinic. Five years from now, I'm not sure, but maybe I'll work part-time in nursing and part-time in business.

My career has been more or less planned, although I have often gone on my gut feeling to determine the best option. I decided that I wanted to continue my education and that I wanted as many options as possible in my life. Since I tend to get bored with endless repetition, I have looked for new challenges often. My current goals and my five-year goals are to teach and to do nursing research. I expect that I will continue to focus much of my research on critical examinations of the medical institution, issues related to nursing's potential role to create needed change, informed consent, client empowerment, high-tech medicine, and death postponement. I expect to develop seminars to teach practicing nurses how to use research methods to improve bedside care and to change work conditions. I will ultimately go independent. It is doubtful that I will work as many hours at critical care nursing five years from now, although I expect to continue doing some critical care in the future. I hated middle-management nursing when I tried it, so it is doubtful that I will seek such a position in the future.

M. Vrtis

I am not career planning. I already know that I will continue with my present author and editor responsibilities and plan to do just that. Concurrently, I will be starting a doctoral program in nursing education.

I achieved my current goals by accepting the challenge to publish. Once my first book was completed, I went on to edit a textbook. Soon after, I was invited to edit a nursing journal. You might say that my success is a combination of hard work coupled with my ability to accept each challenge.

In five years, I plan to be teaching full-time and attending to my journal and publications part-time.

Mary Ellen Luczun

I have only begun to plan my career or contemplate my goals in five years. I hope to become a family nurse practitioner and to work in a rural area five years from now.

G. Berkram

Five year plan? I was never good at those and am probably worse now. I now use tarot cards, astrologers, and hypnotic pseudoorientation in time. I think it works better.

D. Webster

CAREER PLANNING

The concept of a career has changed over the years. In *The Organization Man*, published in 1957, a successful career person was one who worked with one company, accepted its values, and moved up the hierarchy to some supreme position before retiring after a long and successful tenure.

Today, a career is viewed more broadly. Successful moving *up* an organizational hierarchy is not the only measurement of success. Indeed with the development of matrix organizations, moving up may not even be appropriate to career advancement. Lifestyle, meaningfulness of work, personal rewards, as well as money and place in the organization define a career. Certainly, for nurses a broader definition of career is required. We have worked very hard to have career ladders, to keep successful nurses at the bedside, and not to have success equated with moving *up* the hierarchy. Also, as women, our career paths will most likely be punctuated by child birth and some time away from the job (Brooks, 1984; Fitzgerald & Crites, 1980). It is for these reasons that I like the broad definition of career offered by Hall and to which I will orient this discussion:

> . . . the individually perceived sequence of attitudes and behaviors associated with work-related experiences and activities over the span of the person's life. (p. 4)

This definition allows the individual, you and me, to determine what career success means. It also allows homemaking to be considered a career because it does not require that the work take place in a business organization. While the focus of this book is on careers in the organization, I would not want to suggest that such employment is the only valuable one for a nurse.

Career Stages

Careers, like most developmental phenomena, go through stages. The stages can be outlined by simply stating that there is a beginning, a middle, and an end. The beginning is characterized by newness. The place is new; the skills are untried; reality shock occurs; everyone else seems to know what they are doing. It is a scary time, but an important time to assess and learn where you want to be. The first job may be a "bummer" or a false start, or a launching pad for the future.

My first job was being part of a team that set up one of the first medical cardiac intensive care units in the Midwest. I fell into this job because in those days a baccalaureate degree meant management, even though one was a new graduate. I would never recommend this to anyone today, and indeed most employers would not allow it to happen. It was not bad, primarily because ICUs were so new that no one knew what to do, and at least I had no bad habits to overcome. What I learned in this job was that I am no person to have around technology, but I am fantastic with anxiety! I hated the blips of the EKG machines, but I loved helping clients, staff, and residents work through anxiety. So I went off to pursue a master's degree in psychiatric-mental health nursing.

The best possible outcome for the beginning phase of a career is a commitment to some future direction that is personally challenging and valuable. In our rapidly changing work world, you may change careers a few times. Some of the literature on adult development is suggesting that we have four to five careers over the course of our lives. Each new career may mean new education and it will certainly mean going through the anxiety of being a beginner all over again. Hopefully, each successful career change leads to more ease and less anxiety in making the next change.

The middle phase of a career should be a time of increasing responsibility and expertise. The organization and how it works will not be so mysterious; you may even know a few "secrets." Opportunities to teach and to mentor should be sought. If you reach a plateau mid-phase, or burn out or lose your original motivation or enthusiasm, this phase can be painful for the nurse and employer. Lateral movement may bring one "back to life" professionally, or some direct strategies to remotivate oneself might be called for.

The end stage of a career requires preparation for retirement; learning to manage a less structured life; dealing with decreased responsibilities, and so forth. This book deals predominantly with the beginning stages of a career, realizing that there will undoubtedly be several beginning phases for each of us over our lives.

Assessment

The responses about career planning were one of the few where age of the successful nurse made a difference. The younger nurses were more likely to have used some techniques. It is probable that with so many opportunities available that they have had to develop some goals and priorities. It is also possible that they were applying the nursing process to themselves. Career planning can be similar to the nursing process: assess your current career status and skills, plan where you want to be in some time-frame, implement the plan to achieve your goals, and evaluate the outcome.

There are many fine books on career planning, as well as magazines from assorted counseling groups that persons can refer to as they engage in formal career planning. Works by Bolles (1981, 1985), Sher (1979), Levinson (1978), and Moran (1983) are cited in the References. These are good places to start.

The secret to successful career planning is "know thy self." This might be accomplished through meditation, counseling, reflection with loved ones, or by writing a biography of your life. Moran (1983) recommends that you dig out pictures of yourself at various ages and remember what you were like then. You keep a written record of your response to questions such as: What skills (intellectual, emotional, personal attributes) did I have then? how did I feel? do I still have the skills I had then? what do I have now that I didn't have then?

If you repeat these questions at frequent intervals over the life process, you will develop a biography of success and positive attributes that are the basis for building a successful career. Some people will find this contrived and useless. Rarer still is the person who has kept a journal or diary over most of their life. By whatever means, it is necessary to develop a realistic sense of "who I am."

If you engage in this process, you will undoubtedly discover that there are several "yous": the professional woman, the daughter, the wife, the lover, the mother, the lazy person, the ambitious person, and so forth. That's true! What you want to tease out is the professional you and what strengths and needs for development you have.

Sher (1979) uses wishing and fantasy to get to the question of what you want to do and what assets you have to do it. She has you list 20 things at which you are really good and then use those things to create a fantasy of the environment you would be most effectively functional in. Then you create an ideal day in your life. Sher calls this "stylereach," imagining the style of life you would want. She then takes you through a series of exercises designed to search out your goals and to handle negatives in life (loss of love, job, etc.).

Perhaps her most charming chapter is "Winning Through Timidation, or First Aid for Fear" wherein she offers sensible approaches to manage fear. Fear can take many forms in blocking success. One can take a vacation and put off the activities needed to move in a career; one can set expectations so high that they become unattainable; or one can be immobilized by the fear of making mistakes. The ability to confront the fear, to set reasonable expectations, and to learn from mistakes are basic tools for career advancement.

Bolles (1981) asks you to assess yourself in three major categories: self-management skills, work-content skills, and functional/transferable skills. Self-management skills are essentially personal approaches to others, to time, to environment, to authority, and to the material world. Work-content skills are knowledge, activities, and vocabulary that are specific to working successfully in a particular area. Certainly an ICU nurse has a different vocabulary and knowledge base, and engages in activities different from a nurse who practices in a psychiatric setting.

The most important category is the functional/transferable skills because these are not job-specific. These are basic approaches to information, people, and things, that can be generalized across job categories and work environments; for example the work-content skill of knowing how to work a respirator is something one either can or cannot do. Bolles and Zenoff (1977) relate that these skills, however, are the most important to pinpoint. They developed what they call "the Quick Job-Hunting Map" on which you respond to the following subcategories of functional/ transferable skills:

- Using my hands (operating equipment, fixing things)
- Using my body (exercise, amount of physical activity)
- Using my senses (observing)
- Using words (communication skills)
- Using intuition (imagination, insight, foresight)
- Using numbers (accounting, record keeping)
- Using logic (problem solving)
- Using creativity (inventing, improving)
- Using helpfulness (listening, counseling)
- Using art (poetry, art, music)
- Using leadership behavior (being visible, directing others)
- Using follow-through (attention to details)

In order to use these to assess one's strengths, you can write a paragraph about how each "works" in your current position and in past positions. You can write them down one side of a paper marking items that you have mastered to varying degrees. Again, the goal is a realistic assessment of what positive resources you already possess to move forward with a career.

Because of my background as a family therapist, I find the genogram helpful in assessing career patterns. The genogram was developed by Bowen to trace the multigenerational transmission process of family problems which culminated in whatever emotional disturbance the family may be experiencing (Bowen, 1978; Guerin & Pendagast, 1976; Miller & Winstead-Fry, 1982). However, the genogram can be used to trace more benign processes, such as values, relationships, and roles, which are basic to understanding career choices.

A genogram traces the family process over at least three generations. A genogram is a "roadmap of the family relationship system . . ." (Guerin & Pendagast, 1976, p. 452). Symbols are used to present a picture of the family. The most common symbols used are illustrated in Figure 2.1. To create a genogram, you need a large piece of paper or a chalkboard. A family bible or other family chronology may be useful, as well as living grandmothers, grandfathers, and other family members, from whom you can receive historical information.

A completed genogram is shown in Figure 2.2. The tier labeled 1 represents the grandparental generation; tier 2 is the parental, and tier 3 is the present generation. Children are listed left to right, the oldest at the left and youngest right. The two sets of grandparents were married in 1925 and in 1922; the parents married in 1955; the person who is presently career planning is the oldest daughter at 28.

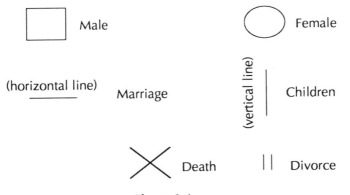

Figure 2.1.
Common genogram symbols.

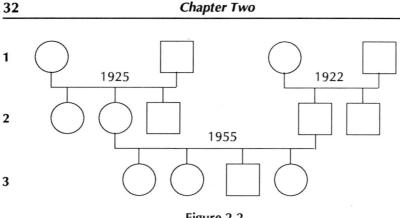

Figure 2.2.
A completed genogram.

In preparing a genogram, you need to pay attention to the roles played by various persons; the values attached to work, love, friendship, and leisure time; what historical events changed the environment of this family? what is the family's reaction to these events (are they a source of pride or of embarrassment)? are there pressures on some members of the family to behave in certain ways? [Boszormenyi-Nagy & Spark (1973) refer to these as "invisible loyalties" that may coerce a family member to fill the dreams or to take the place of a missing family member.] are there stories about successes and failures in the family? do these stories seem congruent with the family history or are they more mythical? do the family values motivate the current generation? are certain vocations valued over others? what is the role of children in the family?

From the genogram should emerge patterns of values, choices, and motivational factors. Figure 2.3 illustrates the completed genogram with the addition of role assignments.

Goal Setting

The next step in career planning is goal setting. It is helpful here to remember that careers go through stages of development from beginning to expert. The stage of one's career may or may not match the rest of one's life. For example, the 40-year-old woman who is suddenly widowed may be a neophyte nurse if she married right after graduation from her baccalaureate program. Simultaneously, in her personal development, she may be at the stages of "intimacy" and "generativity" to use Eric Erikson's scheme (Erikson, 1968). The stage of family development at this moment

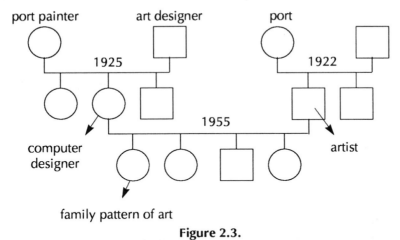

port painter   art designer   port

1925   1922

1955

computer
designer

artist

family pattern of art

Figure 2.3.
Completed genogram with role assignments.

is in crisis due to the death of her spouse. Van Maanen & Schein (1977) offer the idea of the "career cube" to show how development of family, self, and work interact.

A simple career cube is depicted in Figure 2.4.

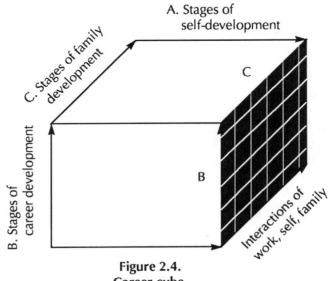

A. Stages of
self-development

C. Stages of family
development

C

B. Stages of
career development

B

Interactions of
work, self, family

Figure 2.4.
Career cube.

The importance of the career cube for our purpose is that career goals be set within the context of what is going on in one's life. Research has shown that women are more likely than men to discuss goals by saying "I hope to ..." Men typically say, "I will ..." or "I plan to ..." (Josefwitz, 1980, p. 67). A goal must be a concrete statement about an action or an event that will occur due to some activity on your part. The statement, "I hope to get a master's degree" might be a fantasy, because hope is not a concrete activity. The statement, "I plan to get a master's degree" is a fact. One can set a date by which the master's will be completed; one can hold oneself accountable for the plan.

Ideally, goals should be written down and a time-frame for achieving them developed. The best goals have the following characteristics:

1. *No* "should" or "ought" statements. Goals say what you *want*.

2. Action verbs: plan, develop, explore, ask, for example.

3. They identify areas that you can influence in fulfilling the goals. If you need money, where can you reasonably get it? No fantasies about winning the lottery are allowed. For example, I have students who have asked their families to forgo a Christmas present and purchase college credits with the money.

4. They are specific about what, when, where, and how the goal is to be achieved.

5. Time-frames for periodic review of the goals.

6. Rewards for achievement of the goal; anything from a candy bar to a mink will do.

7. They are attainable.

I was intrigued that if a particular article or book was written by a woman, the word "attainable" was not used outright to modify goals. It is likely that the career development of women is seen as more varied than that of men; thus that which is attainable at any given time in a woman's life, may be quite variable.

Moran (1983) discusses her observation that women (not specifically nurses) seem to have a harder time setting goals for themselves because they spend so much time being responsible for others: children, aging parents, and spouses. In her experience, few women are comfortable with being totally objective and rational about setting goals. They have to balance personal goals while maintaining healthy, sane familial relationships.

In her study of successful entrepreneurial women, Jennings found that women's goals were stated almost as philosophies with value statements about the product to be produced or sold. I have participated with women trying to achieve goals no one else thought possible. I have seen nurses who did not have the "right" Graduate Record Exam scores, who had no family support for doctoral study, accomplish the PhD. Likewise, I have seen nurses with everything going for them succeed.

At this time, it is probably better if you define "attainable" personally. If you have really assessed your assets and have a realistic picture of who you are, goals should flow from that assessment.

Establishing a timetable for achieving goals involves common sense. To date, we cannot bilocate; so if you have to be in school or at a meeting, or if you have children, you are going to have to make special arrangements. You can delegate some meetings to others, or opt to miss a class or two. But by and large, if you have children, a good baby sitter is a treasure.

Implementing the Career Plan

Once goals have been established, developing a timetable and implementing the plan requires some research and networking. Suppose your goal is to be a head nurse in five years. Assuming there are several employers in the community, you would need to talk to colleagues to find out which employer might have vacancies in five years. This may help you decide where to work (unless, of course, the institution has a pattern of hiring head nurses from the outside). The goal would also most likely require that you take an assistant head nurse job at some time. Are these available? Where? What are the requirements for this position? Obviously, you cannot learn all you need to accomplish the goal of being a head nurse in isolation. Participation in professional organizations, networking with colleagues, and reading local newspapers and relevant professional journals are requisite to accomplishing this goal. A mentor who is a head nurse may also help. Such a person could point you in the right direction and speak of your qualifications within the institution. You can't do it alone!

Once your career plan is implemented, it needs "watering" like any seedling. I sometimes think once a plan is announced, a special gremlin makes sure that anything that can go wrong, does: aging parents get sick, kids come down with the measles on the most important day of the year, and your spouse (if you have one) has to go out of town. There is only one way to deal with these vagaries, and that is to develop a sense of humor.

The other side of the gremlin events is what Jung (1973) called "synchronicity", the apparently spontaneous happening of events that complement one another. I have had more than one student besieged by the gremlin, who may run into a woman waiting on line at the grocery store, who just happens to have the books a student needs and can't get to the library to take out. Relaxing during times of crisis and apparent chaos is not learned easily, but it does seem to open the door to opportunities. It is helpful to remember that the Chinese character for crisis is made up of the characters for *danger* and *opportunity*. Generally, the opportunity comes in the person of someone from your network or family who can provide the margin of relief that gets you through.

Finally, to implement your career plan, I find it helpful to have heroes/heroines to whom you can look. Some persons find these in religious belief; they may be "called" to do whatever it is that they are doing. Some use mythical figures such as the goddesses to inspire them. Therese Connell Meehan's (Connell, 1983) article on feminine consciousness in nursing and Jean Shinoda Bolen's (1984) ideas about goddesses existing in every woman are often helpful. These works are listed in the References.

My own heroes are men: Generals Patton and Rommell. Both attacked enemy shores, invading hostile territory and building their supply lines in the process. This sounds like the life of a working mother to me. Actually, I think Patton and Rommell had it easy. They had the war machines of the United States and Nazi Germany backing them; they had well-trained soldiers and reasonably competent managers; they did not have sick children, arthritic dogs, and husbands with conflicting schedules to deal with. There are days when I envy Patton and the relative simplicity of the Battle of the Bulge!

Intuition

The successful nurses' responses to the role of intuition in career planning were predictably mixed. Successful women seem to combine an intuitive approach to career management with a rational one. Jennings' (1987) study of female entrepreneurs cites Randy Fields, the husband of Debbie Fields, president of Mrs. Fields'® Cookies: he states, "The major feature of a good entrepreneur is terrific intuition." Jennings goes on to discuss how

Fields' soft, chewy cookie violated the market wisdom of crisp cookies. Debbie Fields knew her idea would sell, and it has!

It is difficult to discuss the idea of intuition because some feminists assert that its unscientific nature is reason to discount it, and thus discount women if they are perceived as dependent upon it; some traditional women use "intuition" as a reason to avoid education. I have met very few nurses who do not value something akin to intuition. Almost every experienced nurse whom I have ever talked with can relate stories of moving the emergency cart, almost unconsciously, over to a patient's room, only to have the patient go into cardiac arrest during their shift. Nurses term this phenomenon "intuition," "experience," "finely honed clinical judgment," or some other term. Intuition will be discussed further in Chapter 4 when I present Ned Herrmann's work on cognition; he clearly includes intuition as an aspect of his "creative brain."

PART TWO

Resources for
Career Advancement

Risk Taking

3

I believe that a woman who wants to succeed in a man's world must be a risk taker. I come from a family-training background wherein a woman is secondary to a man and that it is a "woman's job" to make a man happy. As I got older and matured, I changed my thoughts on womanhood and realized that I did not like the role model as displayed by my grandmother. I began to think and function as an equal to men. I believe that women ask permission too often. I work from a design of "do it," and if I am questioned later, I explain my rationale. However, before I take a risk, I assess the situation and decide whether it is worth sticking my neck out for. The criteria for taking a risk for me are

1. Will it benefit the client and does the client want or need it?

2. Will it benefit me and do I really want or need it?

3. Will it benefit a friend (relative) and do they really want it or need it? If the answer to any one of these is yes, then, unequivocally, I take the risk.

A. Clayman

I don't really view myself as a risk taker. To me, a risk taker is one who leaps over tall buildings. I suppose, looking back, I could say that I took a risk when I decided to go back to school after 12 years not practicing nursing. I don't know that I developed risk-taking skills. I just formulated my goal and did what I had to do to achieve it.

Risk taking or not afraid to be unconventional? In high school I had a wide variety of friends. Some of the "in crowd" as well as the fringe group and everything in between. I was the first in my family of five

41

sisters and three brothers to graduate from college; the only girl to have a career. I had to defy my father to attend the large state university. It would have been okay to have attended the Catholic, all-girls college or to have enrolled in a hospital nursing program. I am the only girl in my family to marry a non-Catholic. It all seems so silly now, but then these were big risks. I am the only girl to work while raising a family and the only woman in our neighborhood to work full-time at a profession.

M. Sprik

I wrote a training grant for a graduate concentration in women's health the first year after I received my doctorate in nursing. My new division head (we had about one new one every year at that point) assured me that it was not a good idea, and that to become political was unwise. Sometimes I wish I had followed her advice, but I would not have wanted to miss the opportunity to work with the faculty, students, and consultants on that project. It was a very exciting time for me and I miss the continued stimulation of those trying to put feminist philosophy into practice. I do not miss being a walking target. Feminism is very much the way of life here at the University of Colorado, but it was a dirty word at the University of Illinois. I don't know how much of that was just bad timing, identification by the aggressor, or just plain homophobia. To declare that one sees women as worthy of attention seems to be considerably more controversial than working with the elderly, kids, or working at the VA.

I have no advice to give about risk taking. I am trying to age gracefully, but I have a big mouth and it sometimes ruffles feathers. I like to make people laugh, and sometimes I am imprudent in my choice of subjects, timing, or someone else's sense of reverence. I would like to think that I have seldom created damage to other people. I would also like to think that I have created considerable damage to assumptive frameworks that value money, status, or power over compassion, caring, and honesty. I have become increasingly confused about what's important for me in terms of safety. The more I give up what appears to be safety (or more accurately have it wrenched from my grasp), the less important it seems. My children are grown, my assets are dwindling, and increasingly I have less to lose.

D. Webster

For me, the biggest risk was my acceptance of a position with a small R & E firm that managed a federal grant to provide health care services using teams of nurse practitioners, social workers, and community health nurses to perform outreach programs for the homeless. I have never worked for "soft money" before, and with funding always dubious, this has been as daring as I have been. It seemed appropriate, however, because I would have the opportunity to expand my skills, professional contacts, and opportunities. And I have been able to maximize them! Perhaps I have always known how to network and sell myself and my talents, and fortunately, homelessness is a hot topic right now. I had similar talents before, but working nights as a clinical supervisor, it was hard to "make a splash." Now I am the nurse executive of the only urban program that attends to these critical issues and in some ways I control access to a population that nurses want to help and learn from.

J. Pond

I have always been a risk taker. I have a sign in my office that states the way I feel and look at issues: "The hell I can't buck the system." But before I do that, I do my homework, and ensure that I have an excellent chance of succeeding.

J. Shoup

Risk taking is a skill that has been used to achieve my goals, but it was not necessarily a skill I developed before achieving my goals. It has developed as a result of working toward my goals. Major risks for me have been major job changes or career choices. I started out working on a surgical floor. After two years, I felt that I needed a new challenge, so I transferred to the ICU. I increased the risk by switching to medicine and the medical ICU to broaden my base of experience. After two years there, I decided to return to graduate school and to work part-time in the surgical ICU. Not only was returning to school a risk for my career, but it was a risk financially as well. Recently I accepted a position as a critical-care clinical nurse specialist, a new position at a hospital that has no other clinical nurse specialists at this time. The combined risk for me was a job change and the challenge of developing a new role in a new hospital.

I guess I never thought of myself as a high-risk taker. I usually take quite a while to make a decision. I try to minimize the risks as I see them by evaluating all aspects of the activity, trying to foresee future outcomes of two or three different choices and weighing all of the pros and cons. I also try to learn as much as I can about the potential risk to be taken. Reasonable risks are ones I believe that are necessary and those that I think I need to take, or can take with some potential of success. If it seems the pros outweigh the cons and that the task seems fun and "doable," then I go for it! One thing I always do is ask myself what would I do, or where would I be/not be, or what I would think of myself if I did not make this change. These questions, after all other questions have been asked, help clarify the issues.

R. Brown

Risk taking is a hallmark of my professional life: I went to nursing school when my family did not want me to; I completed my BSN without my family's emotional or financial support; I served in the Peace Corps against family wishes and was a volunteer with the first group to go to Samoa—I was the first PC nurse to teach nursing in that country. From Samoa I applied to graduate school and enrolled in the first MSN program at Wayne State University that educated nurses in expanded practice; I was the first MSN nurse to work for the Detroit VNA and provide direct care to patients and act as a team leader; I was the first nurse with an MSN to work in an expanded practice role in a rural health care setting (they had never hired anyone with an MSN nor anyone who functioned as I did). I became the assistant director of nursing with a director of nursing whose level of education was a diploma.

RISK TAKING

The responses cited here certainly demonstrate that the successful nurses take risks, even though they may not consider themselves risk takers. This is not surprising. Phillippe Petit, who strung a wire between the twin towers of the World Trade Center and walked it, does not consider himself a risk taker! He feels that the hours of practice and planning he does for each walk decreases risk to just about zero (Keyes, 1985).

Although the successful nurses did not respond ambivalently, risk taking is an ambivalent topic for many. There are those who perceive risk taking as a sinful aspect of human nature. For such persons risk taking connotes unnecessary danger and challenging fate. Indeed smoking, excessive alcohol or food consumption, and drug abuse are "risk factors."

The concept of risk in this chapter is often referred to as "psychological" risk. It is not associated with disease, but is associated with growth. Within this view, risk is necessary to be successful within your environment. From infancy on, people take risks to grow. You have only to watch the infant learning to walk to appreciate the necessity and thrill of risk taking. Infants will pull themselves up and fall down repeatedly until the time comes that the infant can stand alone. The face of an infant who has succeeded here is one of the most joyous faces we ever see. The successful nurses reported much the same behavior in adult terms. Taking jobs that they were really not qualified for in their minds, moving to new environments because they felt blocked in their current situation, and creating new roles in nontraditional settings were sources of satisfaction to these women.

Self-Assessment

Self-assessment of your own risk-taking skills requires some self-knowledge. If you are optimistic by nature, it may be hard to see the negative side of situations. You may not perceive risks, only opportunities. If you tend more toward pessimism, slight risks may loom large and you may see opportunities as dangerous.

There is no fool-proof way to assess risk. Conscious risk taking is like creating a mini-crisis in your life. Sometimes risk taking is imposed upon you by the environment. Certainly, the nurses who are providing leadership in the care of AIDS patients never anticipated the risk taking involved in treating these dying, often young persons.

The scale presented in Figure 3.1 was developed by Knowles (1976). It is a quick measure of general risk taking. It is scored as follows:

"Agree very much" and "mildly agree" answers to questions 1, 4, 6, 7, 8, 9, 10, 12, 16, and 18 indicate an unwillingness to take risks. The more "agree very much" answers, the greater the desire to avoid risks. "Mildly disagree" and "disagree very much" answers indicate risk taking. "Neutral" responses indicate that you are not much concerned about these items.

"Agree very much" and "mildly agree" answers to questions 2, 3, 5, 11, 13, 14, 15, 17, 19, and 20 indicate a willingness to take risks. Again, the more "agree very much" answers, the greater the propensity for risk taking. "Mildly disagree" and "disagree very much" answers indicate an unwillingness to take risks. "Neutral" responses indicate not much concern.

COMMON RISKS TAKEN

Divorce

Leaving a "stifling," "empty," "bad" marriage was a risk that was mentioned by some respondents. I did not include any direct quotes regarding divorce because I did not have spouses', usually husbands', permission to cite explicitly personal matters. Husbands were characterized as supportive or

Directions: Below are 20 statements that refer to risky situations. For each statement, indicate how much you agree or disagree by marking the number that most closely corresponds to how you feel about it.

	Agree Very Much	Mildly Agree	Neutral	Mildly Disagree	Disagree Very Much
1. It is always best to look before you leap.	1	2	3	4	5
2. I'm the kind of person who is usually not very cautious.	1	2	3	4	5
3. I enjoy being around people who are willing to take a chance.	1	2	3	4	5
4. I enjoy doing things when I know exactly what is going to happen.	1	2	3	4	5
5. A little recklessness is good for people.	1	2	3	4	5
6. I'm the kind of person who avoids risks.	1	2	3	4	5
7. With the kinds of problems you can run into these days, I'd rather not hitchhike.	1	2	3	4	5
8. I'd rather walk than ride with someone who drives at excessive speeds.	1	2	3	4	5
9. In most situations, it is often better not to take a chance.	1	2	3	4	5
10. I'd rather not gamble if there is some other way of doing things.	1	2	3	4	5
11. I'm the kind of person who enjoys risks.	1	2	3	4	5
12. In most things it is probably better to know exactly what you are doing.	1	2	3	4	5
13. I stay away from situations that are likely to be dangerous.	1	2	3	4	5
14. I tend to like people who have a wild streak in them.	1	2	3	4	5
15. I sometimes gamble just for the excitement it brings.	1	2	3	4	5
16. I'm the kind of person who is usually careful about what she or he does.	1	2	3	4	5
17. I'd rather play with fire than not play at all.	1	2	3	4	5
18. It is better to be safe than sorry.	1	2	3	4	5
19. There is a certain excitement in breaking someone else's rules.	1	2	3	4	5
20. I enjoy getting into situations that I don't know I can get out of.	1	2	3	4	5

Figure 3.1.
The subjective opinion questionnaire.

nonsupportive, especially when it came to wives seeking more education. Several of the women commented that they started back to school without their families' emotional or financial support. Several of these nurses identified themselves as lesbians. However I used traditional, heterosexual marriages when referring to husbands.

From the divorce statistics, the stories in women's journals, and the research done on working wives and mothers, we know that blending a marriage and a career is not easy. It was a surprise that none of the respondents mentioned rotating shifts as a source of dissatisfaction in their marriages. When divorce was mentioned as a risk taken, the reasons offered were always personal growth or an intolerable situation.

Job Change

I insisted on getting a position at this medical center when it first opened, even when the nursing director at that time, who later became my boss for nine years, insisted there were no jobs for me. I persisted in contacting her and applying for anything that became available. She finally hired me into an entry-level management position as a nursing supervisor on the evening shift. The following year she promoted me to the position of director of nursing.

I took a great risk when I came to the hospital. In fact, shortly after my arrival, the medical staff demanded a meeting with the hospital board for the sole purpose of having me terminated. I stood up not only for myself, but for administration, patient care, and my beliefs in what needed to be done at the hospital and in what actions I had taken at that time. The result was that the board upheld my employment and totally changed their perception about our solidarity in approaching the problems both for nursing and for the hospital in general.

Risk taking started out as an interesting concept, and ended up as a real gut-wrenching process during my protracted problems with my hospital. I had stepped over invisible boundaries when I went from being their excellent employee to demanding to be independent as a nurse. The hospital panicked as I think they viewed it as something that might breed anarchy in the other nurses. Most of the other nurses didn't understand how nursing would function outside of the traditional model, and they also viewed me with skepticism.

P. O'Brien

Risk taking is my middle name! I love and dread it at the same time. Creating a new role where one never existed is exciting, but risky. I always seem to put myself into positions for which I am slightly underprepared. For example, the pain nurse specialist role. I knew a lot about behavior techniques with cardiac patients (my MS is in cardiac nursing), but nothing about chronic pain. At first, I just immersed myself in the literature and worked closely with the medical director. Because I had been clear from the start about my competencies, a lag time was expected and supported.

Education

I guess you could call it a risk when I left my comfort zone and ventured into college at the age of 50. It was risk to face all those young people who I was afraid would intimidate me, only to find that it was not that way at all. They were the ages of my own children, and I found that I had their respect rather than their criticism. They would say, "I wish my mom would do something like this."

B. Frampton

I cannot say that I developed risk-taking skills, since they seem to be an innate part of my character as far back as I can remember. I probably have refined those skills over time. I have never been afraid to reach; rather I have learned to carefully evaluate what I am reaching for. Each career decision I have made in nursing has been based on thoughtful evaluation of the costs and benefits of the change. Probably the biggest risk I have taken is the decision I made during my doctoral program to move out of the area of the school, and to take my dissertation with me. I was counseled strongly against this move by the faculty who feared I would never finish. I did not consider this move to be "dangerous," but rather quite reasonable. I knew my limitations and abilities, and completed the dissertation within nine months, while working full-time.

Integrity/Ethical Issues

I believe no job is more important than one's ethics. An example of a risk I took was as a nursing-school chairperson. I had a faculty member who had satisfied criteria for tenure and promotion by her peers, senate committee, and my recommendation. The academic vice president wanted to block her promotion for personal reasons not related to her ability, peer or student relationships, or effectiveness as a nursing faculty member. I took a firm stand that I could not work in an organization that would not honor commitments and offered my resignation. I did not do this flippantly and never did so before or after this episode. The academic vice president consulted with the president, and tenure/promotion was approved, and I did not resign.

K. Bentley

Siegelman (1983) describes three types of risk takers. The anxious risk taker is one who believes there is one correct way to do things and that a reasoned approach will reveal it. Such a person focuses on the possible negative outcomes of the risk and worries about them. Once they have taken the risk, they may wish they had done something else and continue to worry about negative consequences. They do not see the challenge and opportunity in venturing out into the unknown.

The balanced risk taker does not worry. This person completes a reasonable search for alternatives, but stops after obtaining sufficient information. The balanced risk taker realizes that a wrong decision is possible, but not a crisis. Once they have made a decision, they stick to it. This person uses rationality and feelings in assessing the risk, and can appreciate the excitement and the anxiety of decision making.

Finally, Siegelman discusses the careless risk taker. This person loves the excitement of the challenge, but does not tend to think much about alternatives, dangers, and their consequences. They love the action and seldom think about a decision once it is made.

Successful nurses fit the balanced risk taker description, for the most part sounding as if they thought things through carefully, and then did them. When asked about the danger of risks and managing the inherent dangers, there were several strategies for assessing danger and minimizing negative effects of risk taking. In reading the responses, I fantasized that everyone had compared notes, so similar were their responses.

All of the responses reflected some variation of the following principles:

1. Gathering information about the risk

2. Assessing the potential negative and positive consequences of the action

3. Assessing the resources to deal with success or failure

4. Assessing the persons and materials needed to move in the risky direction

5. Planning how to minimize the dangers and maximize the opportunities

6. Planning how to deal with the consequences

These activities match the textbook descriptions of risk-management principles. It is likely that successful people have either developed or intuitively know how to handle risk with both minimal anxiety and minimal carelessness.

In addition to these risk-assessment questions, successful nurses often ask themselves what they would think of themselves if they didn't do this. Keyes (1985), in his discussion of risk taking, says that we often take risks because we don't want to "lose face" in front of others. It seems that the successful nurse respondents do not want to lose face when they examine themselves.

Jennings' (1987) description of successful entrepreneurs puts an interesting twist on conventional literature dealing with risk taking. The women she interviewed never perceived risks because they never entertained the notion of failure! These successful women talked about challenge, opportunity, excitement, and gain and not of fear, chance, danger, or loss. Total absence of a fear of failure may well characterize successful women, regardless of occupation. I did not phrase my survey questions to successful nurses in such a way as to tap this possibility.

EMPOWERMENT

Nursing literature is just beginning to discuss the concept of empowerment. Empowerment suggests an approach to life that includes the power to make choices, to participate in change, and to grow and learn continually. Empowerment is perhaps more descriptive of successful women's experiences than the idea of risk taking because it conveys a sense of inherent self-efficacy and not the notion of a dangerous outside environment often associated with risk taking. Empowered persons do not leap tall buildings; they do live each day with a sense of responsibility and with a sense that anxiety and fear can be managed.

Loughary and Ripley (1977) developed a training program to teach self-empowerment. Self-empowerment means basically that the source of personal power is in the ability of the self to be the locus of control for goal-directed activities. The model assumes that life is probablistically predicable and that one is not controlled to any great extent by unconscious desires or wishes. It assumes that cognition can influence feelings and people can make choices among alternatives. Finally, the model is built upon the idea that people are goal-directed and not manipulated by or helpless in the face of society: People learn to be aware of themselves and to assume responsibility for what they let happen to them. Stress and anxiety are perceived as manageable; they can be observed and dealt with effectively by the self. The person who adopts this view perceives change and transition as the norm, and learns how to set goals and desirable outcomes in the context of a continually changing but manageable society.

Using the conceptual model of nurse Martha E. Rogers, Elizabeth M. Barrett developed the "power as knowing participation in change tool" (PKPCT). Barrett assumes that change is part of life. Sometimes one creates it and other times it comes from outside the self. Risk enters when one creates a change or decides upon a certain course of action in regard to external change. Regardless of the situation, a person who senses that he or she has the ability to knowingly participate in the change will feel differently about the change than one who is a passive recipient of life events.

Both Loughary and Ripley's and Barrett's work are in the beginning stages. Their work deserves watching because it may be more congruous with women's experience of life as a flow of interconnected relationships than risk taking is.

For the present, some of the ideas of power that exist in management literature can supplement our understanding of empowerment. A key element in the move to decentralize organizations is the idea that the locus of decision making and of responsibility/accountability should be at the lowest level possible within the organizational hierarchy. This could be translated to mean that individuals will be empowered to make the decisions that effect their work. It has been established that workers who are acknowledged as expert, create choices, and implement decisions they help make *are* more productive. This is as true, for example, in a Japanese automotive plant, as it is in a nursing-care unit. Part of the attractiveness of primary nursing and other models that allow nurses to practice autonomously is that they fulfill this basic rule of business.

Today, there are many sources of empowerment for nurses. The Diagnostic Related Group (DRG) payment system has put the nursing service department at the forefront of income generation and cost containment. Several recent studies document that a powerful nursing service is related to fewer DRG denials or to enhanced revenues (Fagin, 1986; Punch, 1983; Brooten, et al, 1986).

Increasingly, nurses are on the decision-making boards of national, state, and private health care organizations. Indeed, our historic, and at times naive valuation of caring, is becoming more and more valued as society ages, and cure is not a reasonable goal. Our lobbying groups are seen as effective in state and federal governments.

The "backbone" of nursing has always been patient care. As nurses become more empowered in various settings, new methods for organizing delivery of patient care are emerging. Group practice, primary care, and contract models characterize work places that nurses value. Increasingly, delivery models that nurses value will be used as enticements to attract nurses to employment settings.

Nursing practice is getting further support as researchers are validating practice approaches, actions, and models. Nurses are identifying risk factors and moving to educate or seek legislation to minimize such factors wherever they occur.

Empowerment is based upon a secure sense of self-worth blended with a secure sense of professional worth. Nursing is increasingly characterized by these qualities. The successful nurses demonstrated this combination repeatedly. And finally, too, the economic rewards of a socially valued work are beginning to come to nursing.

4

Decision Making

I am both intuitive and rational in decision making:

Rational	Intuitive
Can I support myself on the salary?	Will this work make me happy/satisfied?
Is there job security?	Do I "fit" into the environment?
Is there an opportunity for growth and advancement?	
Will I be working in a stimulating environment (not doing the same thing every day)?	
Will I have some control over my schedule?	

P. Baumeister

My style of decision making is an integration of heart and head. I am still developing trust in my intuition (we get very little support for this way of decision making!), and believe this is more the way I want to make decisions. My main formula for decision making is how some things feel to me. I do integrate this with looking at my life and deciding intellectually what is realistic and practical for me. I'm not sure I really separate the two, but do lean more heavily on how something feels.

V. Andrus

Decision making is a fairly subjective mechanism. When one is in a position of power, he or she is at liberty to call the shots, so to speak. I can only tell you of my experience as editor. Authors are accountable to me, as well as issue editors. When making decisions, I always *listen* to the concerns and interests of these individuals. Ideas that are feasible are given serious attention. As such, I try to honor certain requests provided they are in keeping with the philosophy of the journal. If this is not the case, however, I politely inform people of the rationale behind my decision. This is the rational component of my decision, but there is definitely an intuitive portion. The intuitive portion inevitably clashes with the rational at times. The possibility of an esoteric topic which I intuitively feel would be appropriate for my journal may not be greeted with the same degree of enthusiasm by my publisher. At times like this, I will be the one to take the risk of convincing the publisher that there is an audience for the subject matter.

Mary Ellen Luczun

[I am] much more intuitive—*not logical*—and I am somewhat rational. My credo in decision making is that I try to have nobody lose. I'll be successful, but *never* at the cost of hurting someone else or not encouraging another to grow.

S. Crandall

I am a rational person and use no set of rules that I am aware of. I try to make business decisions based on return on investment, but also consider the type of activities I most enjoy. I am in a position where I can be self-actualized.

P. Iyer

My decision-making style is both intuitive and rational. I listen carefully to my feelings when I notice a discomfort in my current situation and try to evaluate the causes carefully. I know of my constant need for learning in my work setting. When I feel bored I must expand my knowledge base to increase to my level of satisfaction. I gather a lot of data before making life changes. This period of reflection is important in helping me to make the best decision for me. The most important part of my decision-making is the knowledge that there are *no* perfect decisions. Being willing to make a mistake helps me to accept the consequences of my decisions.

M. Butterfield

I don't think I have a "style" of decision making—although I guess it's more intuitive. I do not have the latitude of moving from the area where I live; so my decisions are made within the context of my community.

I believe that most of the time I like to make decisions by first seeking consultation with others. For instance, if it is important to consider reorganizing a department, I like to talk with key individuals who would be involved, who know the organization very well, who know and are acquainted with other key players, and get their input. In addition, I often discuss large projects with consulting colleagues outside of the organization to again broaden the scope of input. In the final analysis, I make the decision and carry the programs forward. However, I believe that intuitive decision making is important relative to people. Determining who has the right skills for what role, as well as who can be trusted to be loyal not only to me in my leadership role, but to the organization overall is an important judgment.

N. Valentine

I do use a rational approach to decision making, but intuition plays a part too. I trust my own sense.

My style is mostly intuitive and since it has served me well, I shall continue that way. Some career choices have not been options, and while I may have been disappointed, I have a strong religious faith that some better outcome is awaiting me. This has certainly been true. For example, I did not get a position that I really wanted, and that led me to return for nurse-practitioner certification, which led me to this position. I would probably be behind the eight-ball if I had taken that other position (all in retrospect, of course!)

J. Pond

My experience with decision making is that I try to think about it—try to separate the "I feel" from the "I think" and "I believe." If I have difficulty with that, I bounce my ideas off a few trusted and knowledgeable friends and peers. I usually write out the pros and cons. Yes, I am sure I pay attention to the intuitive part of myself. I try to reach a balance between the two (intuitive/rational-logical). This process takes time and I try to "buy time," if I need it.

I am very intuitive, but rational as well. I usually back up my intuition with some input from others or data (whatever is needed). I never make snap judgments.

I use different decision-making styles in different situations. Sometimes I am very "linear" or "left brained," collecting much data and even inventing formulas to weigh options. I always *like* to identify multiple options. Sometimes I select an option intuitively, even when my rational-logical formulas would indicate a different option. If I can find one option, program, action, or whatever, that tends to dovetail to meet all or some of the objectives of various problems at the same time, I am very excited about that. It is usually a very creative decision. When that happens, I always "go for it."

I think I favor rational-logical decision making. I base decisions on clinical, administrative experiences; common sense; application of similar experiences; consultation with other sources. I don't think nurses are truly intuitive. I think they are at a level of expertise where they assimilate information, make decisions, and act so quickly that it *appears* to be intuition, but is actually based on previous knowledge. For administrative or leadership decisions, my style is a flexible one. I am autocratic when staff or situation needs it, i.e., a new graduate needing guidance in an emergency situation. I am democratic when possible. I like input from my staff when it affects unit functioning.

L. Quartararo

DECISION MAKING

In reading the successful nurses' responses, there appears a striking combination of intuition and rational thinking upon which these women comfortably rely. Only a few distinctly preferred one over the other. Certainly, nursing education at the baccalaureate level has stressed critical thinking skills. While many of these women were years ahead of their basic education, it suggests that such skills remain valuable over time.

Brain Lateralization

Recent understanding of the different functions of the left and right brain suggest that persons who can call upon both hemispheres have an advantage. In most people, brain lateralization is characterized by the following pattern: The left brain is primarily responsible for linear thought, writing, mathematical thought, and for speaking. The right brain is responsible for spatial perception, mental-map making, and perception of connections.

Ned Herrmann (1988) considers physiological brain lateralization as a metaphor for how people prefer to process information. He believes that the brain is a whole and that four distinct patterns for conscious knowing can be demonstrated, and that each of these four patterns is associated with certain behavior. He has developed a valid and reliable scale to measure the pattern called the *Herrmann Brain Dominance Instrument* (HBDI). A brief alternative exercise follows. It is not a validated HBDI alternative, but it will give the reader a sense of their preference.

Herrmann offers three caveats in working with the insights gleaned from the scale: (1) Patterns are neither good nor bad, any mode of knowing has its use in some situation; (2) The scale measures *preferences*, not competency. The fact that one has a preference does not make one proficient in performing within the pattern; (3) Patterns tend to remain stable if one's life is stable. The patterns can change or be changed by personal initiative or circumstance.

Self-Assessment Exercise

Without getting into the complex scoring system Herrmann offers, the following summary can guide you in your self-assessment (Figure 4.1): Column A represents thinking processes that are characterized as "fact based," "analytical," "logical," and "quantitative"; Column B represents thinking processes that are characterized as "planned," "detailed," "organized," and "sequential"; Column C represents thinking processes that are characterized as "emotional," "interpersonal," "feeling based," and "kinesthetic"; and Column D represents thinking processes that are characterized as "holistic," "intuitive," "synthesizing," and "integrating" (p. 411).

If you score most in Column A and least in Column C, it would suggest that you prefer a logical, factual approach to decision making to an emotional and interpersonal approach (Figure 4.2). Do note that everyone scores some points in each category (unless you scored every C choice as zero). So your score does not suggest that you are cold and unemotional, but that you *prefer* facts. Remember also, that while this may be your preference, it does not mean that you are good at it. Indeed, if accumulating facts and organizing them logically is your preference and you are not good at doing this, it may be a source of frustration.

As one more example, if you score high in Columns A and D, your profile is similar to what I would infer as being the profile of many of the successful nurses; that is, they score high in both the logical, analytical, and in the holistic, intuitive processes.

This exercise contains four sets of dichotic word pairs. For each set, review the 13 dichotic pairs on the basis of your general preference for one or the other. Indicate your degree of preference for each of the two by dividing 100 points between them as illustrated in this example.

Example:

A–D Dichotic Pairs

Analytic <u>30</u> / <u>70</u> Holistic

Force a choice between all 13 pairs in each set. In doing so, try to avoid a 50/50 split.

After completing all four sets, add up the totals in each column (A, B, C, D). Since all four columns are involved twice, you end up with two totals for each column. Enter these totals below, and determine a grand total for each column. Then write <u>most</u> in the box under the column (A, B, C, D) with the highest total. (If there is a tie, write <u>most</u> in both boxes.) Write <u>least</u> in the box below the section(s) containing the lowest total(s), and <u>some</u> in the boxes under the remaining sections.

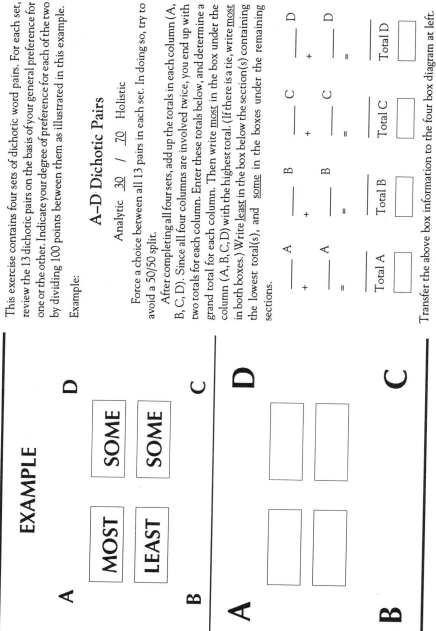

EXAMPLE

A   D

| MOST | SOME |
| LEAST | SOME |

B   C

___ A   ___ B   ___ C   ___ D
+   +   +   +
___ A   ___ B   ___ C   ___ D
=   =   =   =

Total A   Total B   Total C   Total D

A   D

B   C

Transfer the above box information to the four box diagram at left.

A–D Dichotic Pairs

A		D
Analytic	/	Holistic
Argument	/	Experience
Rational	/	Intuitive
Digital	/	Analogue
Explicit	/	Tacit
Analytic	/	Gestalt
Focal	/	Diffuse
Logical	/	Impetuous
Directive	/	Reflective
Words	/	Images
Realistic	/	Imaginative
Factual	/	Metaphoric
Literal	/	Approximate
Total A	/	Total D

B–D Dichotic Pairs

B		D
Detailed	/	Holistic
Sequential	/	Flexible
Safekeeping	/	Experimental
Rule Maker	/	Rule Breaker
Avoids		Accepts
Ambiguity	/	Ambiguity
Evaluative	/	Nonjudgmental
Disciplined	/	Playful
Execution	/	Conception
Planned	/	Impulsive
Structured	/	Free Flow
Controlled	/	Open
Operational	/	Strategic
Organized	/	Nonorganized
Total B	/	Total D

Figure 4.1.
Self-assessment based on dichotic pairs.

Figure 4.1. (continued)

B–C Dichotic Pairs

	B	C	
Verifies	___	___	Feels
Controlled	___	___	Emotional
Implements	___	___	Performs
Procedural	___	___	Free Form
Hard	___	___	Soft
Form	___	___	Feeling
Organization	___	___	Relationships
Dominate	___	___	Accommodate
Sequential	___	___	Harmonious
Dogmatic	___	___	Spiritual
Conservative	___	___	Charitable
Articulates	___	___	Talks
Detailed	___	___	Approximate
Total B	___	___	Total C

A–C Dichotic Pairs

	A	C	
Informational	___	___	Interpersonal
High-Tech	___	___	High-Touch
Intellectual	___	___	Sensuous
Here and Now	___	___	Eternity
Active	___	___	Receptive
Objective	___	___	Subjective
Analytic	___	___	Intuitive
Words	___	___	Music
Worldly	___	___	Spiritual
Facts	___	___	Feelings
Knows	___	___	Senses
Things	___	___	People
Rational	___	___	Emotional
Total A	___	___	Total C

Ways of Knowing

How you make decisions is intimately linked with how you know the world. How women know is a subject that is beginning to be addressed by scholars. One of the better attempts at understanding how women know is presented in *Women's Ways of Knowing* (Belenky, Clinchy, Goldberger, & Tarule, 1986). Belenky and her colleagues studied women from diverse age, socioeconomic, and educational backgrounds; their sample comprised unwed, teenage mothers to doctorally prepared women. These women were interviewed over several years, and their ways of knowing were categorized from the data. They grouped the data into five epistemological categories: silence, received knowledge, subjective knowledge, procedural knowledge, and constructed knowledge (p. 15). They neither posit that these are stages nor does their data allow them to draw conclusions about how women move from one stage to another. The researchers were particularly sensitive to the context of the women's lives and to the problems that each was trying to solve. A brief review of the five epistemological categories follows.

The category labeled *silence* was fortunately rare. Women in this category while neither literally deaf nor dumb, were unable to use words as tools for connecting with others or with themselves. Hence, the designation "silent." Words were weapons used to diminish people. An argument or "mouthing off" often lead to a beating. Representational thought did not exist for these women. Although none were technically illiterate, they were cut off from society and themselves. Language did not lead to exchange of ideas or a sense of connectedness with another. Language kept others from attacking, if one was lucky. Women in this category were cowed by authority. Their attitude was, "If you're smart, you do what authority says and stay out of trouble." Likewise, these women often tolerated brutal marriages because they wouldn't know how to live if their male partners did not control decision making and take action.

These women have not developed a sense of self. One participant, when asked to describe herself, responded, "I don't know . . . . No one has told me yet what they thought of me" (p. 31). They often grew up in families where one parent was brutal, and the other submissive. They were usually isolated from the larger community, so there were no opportunities for contact with the larger world or other role models. Given their background, and their lack of sense that words convey thoughts and connections, these women typically did poorly at school, often just being passed along in the system until they often ultimately quit. None of the "silent" women were found in college. Some college women had been silent, but they learned and moved beyond this stage.

Women who are characterized by *received knowledge* are a mirror image of their silent sisters. As opposed to words devoid of intellect or thought, their words are sacred. These women learn by listening and believing everything authority says. For some, the birth of a child is what turns them from silent to listening and "knowledge receivers." Childbirth upsets their belief that they are totally helpless. The responsibility to care for a dependent infant pushed some of the women to go to child centers for instruction. They listened and found that they could remember and understand. In some cases, staffs at the centers focused upon the women's competence and praised them. Learning by listening to an expert became a valued experience for these women. This pattern is seen not only in mothers, but also in some young college women who expressed joy in listening to classmates and professors.

These women still have little sense of themselves as active agents in their lives. They take in what others say in a literal sense. They accept reality as black or white, good or bad. When experts disagree, they cannot discern argument. One participant reports that she only reads material from the LaLeche League because any other opinion ruins the reading experience. When asked how they would decide an argument between experts in some area most responded that they would follow the idea that had the most popular support.

When authorities do not behave as expected, these women become confused. Teachers who do not hand out "right" answers, but expect students to argue or present their own views, use "wrong" teaching methods, according to these women: These women value objective, honest knowledge, both from their teachers and their friends. They want to find a climate of acceptance and sense of equality that often allows them to begin to think for themselves.

These women are comfortable with traditional sex roles. Because everything is either-or, ambiguity is not tolerated. These women assume that the simultaneous choice of "self" and "other" would realize something dreadful. They must choose either the "self," or the "other," and usually do choose the "other." They are subordinate listeners and followers. Leadership and self-definition is managed by others. Belenky and her colleagues report the comments of a college freshman: "Everything I say about myself is what other people tell me I am. You get a pretty good idea of yourself from the comments that other people are saying about you" (p. 48).

These women's saving grace is paradoxically that they listen and internalize what they hear. If they encounter a teacher, parole officer, or another who affirms their intelligence and competence, they begin to see themselves in this way. However, they still have a way to go before they perceive themselves as masters of their own fate and in control of their own lives. Both the "silent" and the "received knowledge" women are at a disadvantage in a rapidly changing world because they have no personal "rudder" to steer them through the turbulent times life often presents.

The third epistemological category is what Belenky and her colleagues term the *subjective knowledge* group. Women in this category have learned to listen to themselves. One woman described her way to knowing as, "I can only know with my gut. I've got it tuned to a point where I think and feel all at the same time and I know what is right. My gut is my best friend, the one thing in the world that won't let me down or lie to me or back away from me" (p. 53).

For many of the women studied by Belenky and her colleagues, the emergence of subjective knowledge heralded a shift from a passive, authority-oriented life-style to one in which women felt more in control. These women often were able to leave abusive husbands, sometimes with small children, and venture to find a life for themselves with little in the way of outside support. This form of knowledge is still dualistic in that there is a rigid approach to right and wrong answers. Now, right answers reside only within the self, and wrong answers with the books, experts, and parents.

Unlike the theories of development posited by Piaget (1952), Erikson (1968), and Kohlberg (1969), which state that the shift from an external authoritarianism to a more inward directedness occurs in adolescence, Belenky and colleagues' research found the shift occurring " . . . from 16 to 60" (p. 54). Regardless of age, the women found this experience exhilarating and freeing. The authors believe this is " . . . an important adaptive move in the service of self-protection, self-assertion, and self-definition. Women become their own authorities" (p. 54). While subjectivism might be seen as stereotypically "female intuition," there were strengths associated with it for these women. It also needs to be remembered that in Eastern thought, and in Western thought until the 19th century, intuition was the primary way of knowing, and for some, the *only* way to know God.

Subjective thought often began after the males on whom the women were dependent failed them, through either abuse or death. Regardless of that initial trauma, educational background, socioeconomic status, or age, the result was a deepened sense of self and a sense of where to go in the world. At this point, the women began to turn to "maternal figures," whether in the form of a mother, a sensitive boyfriend, or a benign social agency. They began to share ideas and experiences and found that they had something of value inside themselves.

The authors describe the liberation of this experience:

> The discovery that firsthand experience is a valuable source of knowledge emerges again and again in the stories of subjectivist women. Suddenly all they experienced in the course of living takes on new meaning—pleasing others sensitized them to people's moods and needs, placating family members or close friends taught them much about negotiation and groups, managing households taught them organizational and financial skills, raising children taught them about growth, health, and illness. (p. 61)

Another group of women who become subjectivists are those the researchers call "hidden multiplists." These women come from backgrounds rich with advantages. However, they were not encouraged, as their brothers were, to become independent thinkers. These women do not suffer the physical problems of abuse that their subjectivist sisters do, but they do suffer isolation and alienation. They develop unorthodox beliefs that they do not communicate out loud. They may tell friends or write poetry about their ideas. They often have a hard time in school because they are rebels at heart. Because they do not discuss their beliefs, some never find a mentor.

The subjectivist position, while personally enhancing for the woman, can be a problem in education and work settings where some adherence to outside standards is required. Some of these women play along and satisfy the standards while distrusting and even hating the rational approach to life. Some of them return to school where they may have difficulty with sciences and other subjects that require logic. Some become very angry at what they perceive as the male orientation of most of society and balk at ever having to conform.

The move to a subjectivist position often involves a dramatic break with the past: leaving home or an abusive husband. As might be expected in such circumstances, the sense of self is in flux. From being the good girls who took care of everyone and accepted the authority of others, these women throw this identity away. Often a new sense of self has a hard time emerging. Regardless of the women's age upon entering this period in life, images of rebirth, childhood, and new beginnings were often cited as dominant themes. They have not yet learned to speak out and to generalize from their experiences, but many were on the way.

The fourth category of knowledge the researchers describe is *procedural knowledge*, the beginning of rational thought. The women who demonstrated this kind of knowing were not born with it. Many arrived through the pain and problems created by subjective knowing. If all knowledge is subjective, what right do parents have to set limits? What right do teachers have to grade students? These questions and the fact that there were teachers and parents impinging upon one's subjective approach to life led to conflict. The difference in the development of these women seems to be that the authorities were benign, or at least meant well. The parents were not abusive, the teachers were not tyrants. They were performing their roles as best they could. This created an atmosphere where listening to others was possible.

Belenky and her colleagues report the story of one young woman, Patti, who took her parents for counseling, assuming that the counselor would be on her side. The counselor was on everyone's side and for the first time, Patti listened to her parents. While Patti was caught in subjectivism, her parents' views were irrelevant. Once she began to listen to them, she discovered that they were people who were also struggling with how to live (pp. 88–90).

These researchers write that formal education seems to be essential to this step. The case of Patti and her counselor was the only one in which formal education did not play a role in the achievement of rational thought and the ability to voice it.

The state of procedural knowledge is not a comfortable situation. Women in this epistemological state lack the assurance that "received knowledge" and "subjective knowers" have. Thinking and listening to and with others is risky. One might be wrong. Others who listen to you might be critical, and there are always complexities in the world. Such women become temporarily quiet as they attempt to learn the skills needed to obtain and communicate knowledge. They can become obsessed with method. It is almost as if the question does not matter, just so one reasons it correctly. However, learning the procedures for analyzing and understanding the world make it a more manageable place. Perspective taking, understanding where others are coming from, becomes a challenge.

Within the rubric of procedural knowledge, two forms of knowing emerged which the authors labeled "separate knowing" and "connected knowing" (p. 101), borrowing the terms from Gilligan (1982). Separate knowers are interested in themselves and the rules that guide knowing from a distance. Often they were tomboys who continue to refuse conventional female roles, and address the world from the view of an impersonal reason. They have a dislike for any idea that "feels right." While they can construct arguments, they generally only do so at the behest of authorities, for example, teachers. Few like to argue among themselves or in the dormitory. Getting too emotional is perceived as "typically female" and not valued.

Connected knowers, on the other hand, are characterized by empathy. They can learn by the experience of others. They move from learning the facts of another's life to learning how the other thinks. They are connected to the object of their knowledge. They try to imagine themselves in the shoes of the person they are trying to learn. They genuinely care about the object of their attention be it a person or a poem.

Both types of procedural knowers, however, are seeking a more objective approach to learning, an approach that separates them from the object of their interest. They are still enmeshed in the system and do not question the basic assumptions of the situation. For example, if a procedural knower becomes a feminist, she will want equality within the economic system that exists. She will not question the value of the economic system. These women move on to the next epistemological state, *constructed knowledge*, after they take some time out and begin to question some of the procedures they were taught. Some separate knowers may take a year off to find the pattern of their uniqueness. Connected knowers talk more about finding missing or lost parts of themselves. Both groups are still not yet integrated persons who blend different modes of thought or question the world to which they are exposed.

The fifth epistemological state the researchers described was that of *constructed knowledge*. Women in this category tolerate ambiguity. They want to deal with all the complexities of life and not compartmentalize them into work and home, thought and feeling, and so on. Their basic premise is that "all knowledge is constructed, and the knower is an intimate part of the known" (p. 137). They understand that knowledge is embedded in a cultural-historical matrix and that it is relative. This is freeing and allows them to explore questions and answers from a variety of perspectives. Because the road to understanding is always under construction, these women become passionate learners.

The tendency of the connected learner to care about a subject can become actually painful for the constructed knower. Their empathic connectedness can lead them to identify with the pain and sadness of women with whom they have enormous differences. "Attentive caring" (p. 142) allows these women to communicate with persons and ideas. They use the language of connectedness to describe their work. Belenky and her colleagues cite the Nobel laureate Barbara McClintock, whose work deals with corn genetics. McClintock says, "I know them [the corn] intimately and I find it a great pleasure to know them" (1983, p. 198). She listens to what the corn has to say and could write a biography about each corn plant. Certainly, a different way to describe how one goes about science!

Constructed knowers differentiate "real talk" from other talk. Real talk comprises a genuine interest on the part of the speaker to share ideas; it requires deep listening. For these women listening is not a passive activity (as it was in received knowledge), but a challenge to share the self with the other. These women can experience pain if they are in a situation where women are expected to be silent or not too bright. Sometimes they cave in, knowing that the world will not change overnight. At other times they may quit intimate relationships or change jobs.

More than any other group of women in the study, these women had a sense of life as foreseen. They questioned and planned to merge family, children, and job with recreation, social concerns, and other important issues. They saw their lives, like their knowledge, constructed from many aspects by themselves. They were not superwomen and did compromise and balance what seemed feasible at some given time.

Their comfort in listening, seeking input from others, weighing pros and cons, and using intuition suggests that successful nurses are in the connected-knower or constructed-knower epistemological categories. This state also characterized successful women in other business ventures (Jennings, 1987; Moran, 1983).

BEST DECISION

When asked about the best decision made to date, the successful nurses were practically of one voice in responding with education. The following quotations are representative of their responses. I have included the quotations from persons who provided different answers because they are good examples of self-confident decision.

> [My] best decision thus far was to go back to graduate school in nursing. It exposed me to a whole new world in nursing, and to a new view of myself as a nurse.

I don't think I have "one best decision." Success is built on a consistent track record of more good decisions than bad and the ability to recognize the bad ones and correct the course at that point.

The best decision I have made career-wise was to return to school. I am nearly finished with my master's in nursing administration.

The best decision I made in my career was a realization that I had skills that not all other nurses had. If I was to make a *difference*, I needed to lead others. Thus, I broke away from the traditional staff nurse role.

J. Steele

The best decision I have made about my career was getting a master's degree.

The best decision I made was to pursue a doctorate. The best thing that happened to me was to marry my husband (of 21 years) who has supported me all of the way. The next best thing was to come to work at my current institution under my current boss.

The best decision I've made was to be the driving force and lead author of our first book. That experience and exposure was rewarding in ways far beyond royalty checks.

P. Iyer

My best decision was to continue to go to school. I quit nursing school after one year in 1960 and got married. I went back to nursing school in 1962, got pregnant, but kept going. I graduated with my diploma in 1967. In 1967, with two kids, I started my BSN. I completed it in 1971, with another baby. Now with three kids, I did graduate school from 1973–1975. The nurse practitioner program was a very wise career-business choice because it made me a generalist who can practice widely or narrowly as opportunity permits.

S. Crandall

The best decision I've made was to come to the University of Washington for my PhD when I did. Great choice and great timing!

K. Allman

The implications of these "best decisions" will be referred to later, in Chapter 5, because so many of the decisions involved education.

Education

Formal education has by far been the most successful career advancer.

J. Shoup

The greatest tool has been formal education. The effect of continuing education has been minimal.

Graduate school was a major tool for career advancement. There is minimal opportunity for independent practice without a master's. Informal education has facilitated obtaining certification, but has had no direct influence on my career to date.

B. Robbins

Formal education has provided me with a breadth of clinical exposure. At my master's program, I was exposed to family therapy, psychophysiologic principles of treatment and micro-teaching elements. All of these interested me. Later, I could use all the interests in my professional work. Continuing education was useful in expanding my skill level for a specific purpose, for example, child development classes at the psychoanalytic institute when I worked with children, and quality assurance classes when I was responsible for developing a quality assurance program as an administrator in a community mental health center.

M. Butterfield

Formal education via the baccalaureate degree was the ticket for the opening of doors for me. Continuing education enhances and reinforces my original educational foundation. My basic four-year degree was the strongest link for my success. Within this program existed nurses who were in private practice, nurses who were leaders (Lucille Joel and Dorothy DeMaio), and nurses who cared about people and nursing. With this type of education, I do not believe anyone could fail.

A. Clayman, New Jersey, NA

The best tool for career advancement has been my ability to apply formal education in informal contexts. I value informal education almost more than formal education because I determine its value and content, but I realize the BS, MS, and CNM are essential credentials.

M. Scoville

I am a firm believer in formal education as a major tool for career advancement. I do not believe that one can simply learn "on the job," although there are many talented people who can progress beyond their earliest expectations without a formal education. I do not understand why so many nurses discount the value of a formal education. I think that the foundation that a formal education provides gives one a base for assessing other opportunities that can then best be met through informal or continuing-education experiences. I do not feel that I would have had the personal confidence, nor the knowledge base to have progressed as rapidly as I did if I had not had the formal undergraduate and graduate educational experiences that I have had the opportunity to pursue.

N. Valentine

Formal education, I think, has played a minor part in career advancements, except for the fact that it is necessary to have a master's degree. Informal and continuing education has taught me more. On-the-job training has taught me more than I ever learned in any classroom since I have gone through my diploma program. I believe that my basic diploma program was absolutely superior to many programs of other individuals, and armed me extremely well for many, many years with regard to my own discipline and my understanding of the fundamentals of nursing which I continue to apply as I administer the hospital.

My PhD was a "door opener." After that, it was up to me. But it was just what I needed. It helped me achieve credibility, and then my own abilities could be recognized and used. I do not have a master's in nursing, but the only area that has really been a limiting factor in is academia, which I'm not concerned about. I have an excellent research background and can hold my own with the best!

Receiving my MS has enabled me to understand many things better (group process, management, etc.). It also was needed to uphold my reputation since I lecture to health care professionals with advanced degrees.

I. Deininger

Formal education has been *the* tool for career advancement for me. Continuing education has been a tool for advancement in terms of becoming and staying certified by the American Nurses' Association. Continuing education fires my enthusiasm, keeps me current, etc. This helps when interviewing for jobs.

Formal education has been a tool in that it has opened doors for the external or outer aspects of my career. I have found it to be personally an obstacle in expressing all that I am because it is so mind-oriented and outer-focused. The truth cannot be found "out there"; it is inside.

S. Reusch

I believe my degrees have secured my advancement. Without them, I would have had to prove my abilities even more significantly in order to be given a chance at higher-level positions. I would not have been given the opportunity to be a nursing administrator with a BSN. The [Joint Commission for the Accreditation of Hospitals Organization] JCAHO requires more in the standards for nursing service. The organization would not have elevated me to associate hospital administrator status without a master's degree because it is an organizational standard for the role. There are other higher-level positions in this system, such as human resource director (a senior manager) which have been filled by candidates with bachelor degrees. In the last 14 years, both incumbents were internal candidates who had risen through the ranks. The competition is stiff in large organizations for higher-level management positions. The edge you get is by a proven track record within the system (internal applicants always have the edge), or by appropriate degrees and other related credentials, if you are an external candidate.

I inherited an insatiable (although I'm becoming saturated now) quest for knowledge from my dad. I hope I'm always learning; that's when I'm the happiest. My master's degree legitimized my nurse-practitioner skills. I also gained important concepts and skills for leadership, organization, writing, research, etc. My PhD studies added breadth and depth to research, conceptualizing, etc. I always contend that formal education gives me confidence in myself, foremost. Sort of like the Wizard of Oz giving courage to the Cowardly Lion.

M. Sprik

Formal education was mandatory for my advancement. I would not be where I am now without it. No ifs, ands, or buts. I find it also important to be involved with a variety of other organizations: Sigma Theta Tau, [American Nurses' Association/Pennsylvania Nurses' Association] ANA/PNA, [Nurses' Association of the American College of Obstetricians and Gynecologists] NAACOG, and, believe it or not, the Junior League. I can make a real statement there for professional nursing.

J. Pond

[A] PhD opens many doors, particularly in nursing education. Continuing education has not provided career advancement for the most part, but provided for personal growth needs.

K. Bentley

Education has made the difference in my life because it helped me stretch myself.

S. Crandall

Graduate school was inevitable. In my current practice, the MS is really entry-level. I am impatient with the continuing debate among nurses regarding entry level at the BSN level. We are not keeping up with other disciplines; entry level for many of them is graduate school.

Formal education is important. The initials [of a degree] will give me more opportunities. Informal/continuing education has given me tastes of new concepts which may have been of interest. Some I have followed up on and further expanded my knowledge.

P. Connelly

Education has been my key to success, the basic foundation for the career that I was to build. Leadership was not always easy for me, but education, experience, risk taking, and a little maturity has made it not only easier, but something I actively seek.

D. Quinn

Advanced formal education has been the cornerstone of my career advancement. Because I knew I wanted an extended clinical role as a nurse-midwife, formal education was the only means to that goal. Informal and continuing education have been more for personal interest and for enrichment peripheral to my career goals.

Formal education has been a major factor in my career. I have participated in continuing-education programs which have assisted me as well, but I don't believe I would be where I am today without my education and guidance from the University of Pennsylvania.

E. Chapman

[A] BSN has been a very important tool. Informal education "planted seeds" for growth. It stimulated interest in moving out of the traditional hospital setting.

From my perspective, the BScN did not advance my career. I was encouraged to take a supervisory role, which I did, but I was not an administrator. This was a wrong career choice for me. I felt more powerless in supervision than as a staff nurse and I always felt torn between doing what I knew was right and what the system demanded.

Returning to practice with an MScN has advanced my career by enhancing autonomy, writing skills, and research and theoretical expertise. These things all contribute to my career advancement.

Informal education has also been critical for my advancement because it validates my role and I learn by being with both patients and colleagues.

G. Mitchell

Continuing education fulfills my goals.

D. Boyle

Formal education has played a part in the attainment of certain jobs, but more than job attainment, my past education affects my job performance. My graduate studies in nursing administration have left me with a definite philosophy of nursing and management. I operate based on these philosophies. Theories that work are wonderful. They allow you to plan, to predict, and to be efficient.

I think if there was any surprise in the responses of the successful nurses, the overwhelming vote of confidence in formal education was it. I can remember over the years, telling students that a master's degree changed one's perception dramatically. Most of my students will remind me of the truth of my assertion when we meet. These successful nurses go beyond my experience. For some the baccalaureate degree was the key; for others the master's or doctorate.

While professionals in nursing have spent more time than most other disciplines debating types of education in regard to role preparation and so forth, the fact that formal education is *the* career advancer in nursing is understood. I have never thought that nurses were a unique subspecies of women, or people who would find rewards and pleasure in some set of social values different from that of the rest of the population. Our society values education; a college education is the norm today; so it is easy to deduce that nurses, as members of society, would value formal education. That education is linked to success is true throughout our society, and holds true for nursing as well.

SELF-ASSESSMENT

The self-assessment for educational adequacy builds directly on the goals developed in Chapter 2. The self-assessment will follow the skill categories Bolles (1981) described: self-management skills, functional/transferable skills, and work-content skills.

Self-Management Skills

You will recall from Chapter 2 that self-management skills are essentially personal approaches to other persons, to time, to the environment, to authority, and to the material world. There is no exhaustive list of these skills, however alertness, commitment to growth, courage, empathy, firmness, flexibility, good judgment, honesty, reliability, tolerance, and a sense of humor are certainly counted among them. [See page 145 of *The Three Boxes of Life* (Bolles, 1981) for a more exhaustive listing.] These skills are learned from relationships with other people, from art and literature, and from interaction with nature and other environments. These skills can be outlined as follows:

1. Relationship skills

    a. Can I listen to another and validate through feedback that I heard what was said? (The negative side of this question is: When listening to another, am I so busy forming my reply that I often do not hear what is said?)

b. Can I laugh at myself? If yes, can I laugh at myself when I am wrong, as well as when I am right?

c. Am I empathetic? Can I take the perspective of another person, even if I don't agree with their actions or beliefs?

d. Am I honest with myself emotionally? Am I honest with others? Am I honest with people's property?

e. Can I "scan" the environment and locate people whom I can help or who can help me? Do I know how to approach people so I can offer them my best and ask for their best?

f. How do I relate to authority? Whatever my style, does it advance my goals?

g. How do I relate to subordinates? Am I respectful? Am I fair?

h. Do I have some method of stress reduction/happiness enhancement, that I practice regularly?

These questions deal with a few of the generic relationship skills needed to be successful. Other skills, such as tact, diplomacy, and so on, are more situation-specific and their value needs to be assessed in the context of the work environment. It is often helpful to form a temporary support group to identify the relationship skills that are necessary for your environment at this moment. If your workplace is emerging from a time of low growth to one of increased productivity, the relationship skills needed to navigate through this time will differ from those needed when maintenance was the goal.

2. Art and literature skills

a. Can I discuss some aspect of the contemporary art or literature scene? Movies? Music? Painting? Books? Television?

b. Do I read the newspaper, magazines, and some nonprofessional materials each week? Each month?

c. Do I have some outlet for my creativity other than work?

d. Can I write a short article that communicates a feeling or an idea about myself?

3. Interaction with nature and other environment skills

a. Is my home reflective of the type of environment that I enjoy and thrive in?

b. Do I "tune into" some aspect of the natural world? Pets? Sunrises or sunsets? Mountains?

c. Where am I most comfortable? Do I go there often enough? What do I get from being there? (This place can be geographically real or an imagined place reached through meditation.)

These are some of the questions that one would want to be satisfied with in order to be satisfied with self-management skills. Obviously, there are no right or wrong answers to these questions. The bottom-line question that determines your success with self-management skills is, "Have work, relationships and play been integrated in a way that is satisfying for me?" The answer to that question will change over time.

Functional/Transferable Skills

As mentioned in Chapter 2, these are the most important skills because they allow one to move among options. Personal-management skills orient one toward life, but they do not necessarily give direction. Compassion is compassion. Honesty is honesty. These can be expressed in just about any setting. In Buddhist thought, one aspect of the path is "right work." The only work Buddha mentioned as wrong was gun running. Any other career can be an outlet for honesty, compassion, tolerance and so forth.

Functional/transferable skills are directed toward three domains: information, people, and things. Bolles (1981) points out that these can be either learned or exist as a "natural" aptitude. For example, the child who is an excellent baseball player will have excellent eye-hand coordination in other areas of work and play. Functional/transferable skills can be outlined as follows:

1. Information skills

a. Can I compare data noting similarities and differences?

b. Can I synthesize material?

c. Can I look at a set of data and discern patterns and opportunities for innovation?

d. Can I organize or compile a group of data into an intelligible whole?

e. Can I accurately copy materials?

f. Can I analyze a set of data, noting the separate parts and their interrelated characteristics?

2. People skills

a. Can I follow instructions accurately and completely?

b. Do I note my activities in the appropriate record?

c. Can I communicate clearly and accurately?

d. Can I teach patients, peers, subordinates, and superordinates effectively?

e. Can I supervise people in such a way that individual and system goals are accomplished?

f. Can I negotiate?

g. Am I at a point where I might be a mentor for others?

3. Thing skills

a. Can I operate the basic machines/appliances that are part of 20th-century life?

b. Can I work a computer? A typewriter? A VCR?

c. Can I integrate high-tech and high-touch?

d. Am I precise in my use of and interpretation of data from machines?

e. Can I manipulate basic nursing technology (e.g., syringes, dressings, etc.) in such a way as to assure patient comfort?

Again, not each of these skills are developed to the same degree by every nurse. Some skills also include others. For example, it would be impossible to synthesize if one could not compare and analyze (Bolles, 1981, p. 147).

Work-Content Skills

Work-content skills are specific to a job. The vocabulary of medicine and nursing is an example. NPO, BID, and so forth, are specific to working in a nursing environment. Engineers do not use this language! It is difficult to design a self-assessment tool for this domain because these skills are so specific to workplace. Certainly, the operating-room nurse has a set of work-content skills different from the community health nurse. The basic assessment question here is "Am I current in the language, the technology, and the value issues of my area of nursing?" To answer this question positively obviously requires attendance in continuing education programs, reading, and feedback from colleagues and clients about the service you provide.

If you look at the vast array of skills needed to manage both career and personal life, it is not surprising that successful nurses value formal nursing education. Some of these skills are inborn, nurtured, and promoted by family life, but all of them can be enhanced and elaborated upon by education.

The baccalaureate degree, which has been rooted in liberal arts since its inception, hones self-management skills by exposing a student to art and literature, as well as the sciences. Because they are inextricably bound to continuity and change, the self-management skills are furthered by a student's participation in birth, death, and the search for meaning that occurs when, for example, a young person is paralyzed in an accident, or a baby is born with a birth defect.

For many, the first lessons in work-content skills come at that level. For nurses who hold associate degrees or diplomas, and are seeking the baccalaureate degree, work-content skills are learned through repetition. The joy of learning how to give injections, read ECG tapes, and so on are part of most nurses' memories of their basic preparation. Baccalaureate education in nursing directly addresses the enhancement of functional/transferable skills by the emphasis placed upon problem solving (nursing process and research), critical thinking, and how to deliver nursing services in multiple settings. Maintaining some form of sterile technique in a single-room-occupancy hotel stretches one's ability to transfer knowledge from one setting to another.

Depending upon your goals and level of professional maturity, continuing education can be instrumental in enhancing any of these skill domains. Certainly, a course in accounting, computers, or executive communication can provide a missing piece needed for career advancement or illuminate new career possibilities. Meditation training, stress management, or a time-management course can enhance self-management skills by offering alternative ways of approaching life. These learnings may be transferred to work-content areas by teaching hypertensive clients to meditate, for example. Sometimes, it is just fun to take a continuing-education course for the sake of learning! I am currently learning Chinese because it is stimulating and gives me something valuable to do on my long commute.

Graduate study at the master's or doctoral level, is also valued by successful nurses. Master's programs generally offer opportunity to enhance work-content skills in a nursing specialty and in a management, teaching, or clinician role. It was clear from the comments of the successful nurses that such preparation went beyond work-content and enhanced self-esteem and other self-management skills. Generally, the doctoral degree offers the nurse in-depth exposure to the rigors of research. The nurses who mentioned this degree always associated it with the goal of a research career.

LOOSE ENDS

Reflecting on the role of education, especially formal education, in these successful nurses' lives, Belenky and her colleagues' research on how women know and how that knowledge influences their actions comes to mind. These nurses are certainly not silent! They write clearly and authoritatively about their experiences and about themselves. Their responses convey a sense of purpose, power, and joy about where they are in life. Even the few who do not like their current positions were optimistic that they would get back to a better place. Belenky and her colleagues also found that college education was essential to moving to an epistemological state in which one has control over and sense of participation in the life process.

Another thought that developed in writing this chapter had to do with depression. Barron McBride, in the Fall 1989 edition of *Reflections*, reported on a study of Sigma Theta Tau members which has not been replicated. However, several of the findings are of interest and may raise important questions that could enhance the emotional functioning of women. McBride reported that the level of depression in her sample was about the national average, 23.7 percent. Furthermore, the level of depression decreased with an increase in the level of education; that is, the higher the education level, the lower the probability of depression. High-level depression was associated with not achieving goals or lack of goals. Perhaps successful career planning is good for one's emotional health!

Another interesting finding is that these women could handle multiple roles (mother, nurse, and so on), as long as the roles were experienced as nonconflicting. This finding becomes more significant when realized in the framework that Belenky and her colleagues developed. The women in the epistemological category of constructed knowledge were not super-women, but were able to compromise and alter their commitments to achieve a feasible balance. The category of constructed knowledge was almost always connected with a college education, or beyond. Would it not be interesting if, for some women, education acted as a buffer against depression? Obviously, this is a speculation at the moment, but it is worth thinking about.

One final thought that may help students make quicker progress toward the baccalaureate degree: When it comes to work-content skills, most baccalaureate programs have some system or challenge exams or credit for life experience for the registered nurse to progress without repeating this learning.

Bolles' (1981) idea that functional/transferable skills are the most mobile skills raises a question about finding a way to validate these skills more systematically than most programs do (in my experience). Josefowitz (1980) discusses the equivalency between homemaker skills and management skills. She provides a two-column comparison of these skills. A couple of examples will illustrate the point.

The homemaker's experience with budgeting for food, clothing, rent, recreation, and so on, is a piece of the managerial function of planning. Negotiation, a managerial skill, is practiced by the homemaker when she bargains a good deal on a car or an appliance. Negotiation is also a part of dealing with service and repair personnel. She practices mediation when dealing with sibling conflict or other family disputes (p. 27).

Assuming that the two primary nursing roles are direct(ing) patient care and integrating the system for the benefit of the patient, his or her family, and co-workers, might it be possible to develop challenge exams for the integration of the system role? Most of the skills needed to implement this role successfully are managerial. If one accepts Josefowitz's logic, and banks and other businesses are doing so more frequently, the development of challenge exams or credit-for-life-experience mechanisms might advance the adult learner to the baccalaureate degree more quickly.

6

Understanding the System

The system I currently work in is the federal government, a megapolitical system. The health-policy work I am engaged in, while nonpartisan and advisory in nature, has tremendous political overtones and undertones. In order to manage the system, one needs to (a) carefully assess the environment into which policy issues are being introduced; (b) target activities that are meaningful and politically relevant; and (c) package them to assure a fair hearing. The nursing system with which I interact is the larger professional organization of nurses for information sharing and introduction of nursing objectives, where possible, into health policy agenda.

I work in a shared-governance model. I try to network with as many departments as possible; so I am not just a name. Being supportive of and open with peers helps.

The system here is rather chaotic and irrational. It is much like being in a third-world setting. Many of the supports required to make a modern system run efficiently are not here. For example, after accepting the nurse-education position, I had to create my own office. I still don't have a phone because the hospital electrician quit and has not been replaced. This system is sometimes better manipulated than managed. To receive the nurse-educator position, I had to quit my staff position and threaten to leave. The system itself is a traditional power-and-authority-at-the-top sort of arrangement. Change comes from the top down, or not at all. This power structure is at times difficult to work with.

I have not found a way to manage the system, but ways to manage myself within systems and organizations. I work in a Catholic hospital where the mission statement of "healing" is, by most, taken to heart. There is an environment of respect, creativity, and self-expression. My immediate boss, the vice president of patient care services, expresses her visions intuitively and this allows others freedom. Risk taking is rewarded on the simple premise that someone tried something. Whether or not it worked completely isn't the issue. When things do not turn out as planned, she asks, "What did we learn and what do we need to do to strengthen it?"

We also have a holistic framework over our nursing practice. This is based on the philosophy of traditional Indian medicine. We have a Department of Traditional Indian Medicine, directed by a medicine man. The conferences he directs are a vehicle for spiritual development. This adds strength to individuals by developing more self-responsibility and accountability. There is a belief in our nursing division that the more accountable one becomes, the more freedom one feels, both for self and in practice. This has most certainly contributed to the creativity I feel in the environment.

S. Rusch

Understanding the system you work within is vital. It is important not to push against it, but to work with it and around it, to be able to move ahead and achieve personal goals. I work as a program director of the State Department of Health. This is an incredible bureaucracy. It has been important for me as a nurse to realize I am part of a team, and a vital part. I have also been willing to be a little nonconformist; a bureaucracy will eat you alive if you let it. A person must be willing to stand up for themselves. One must also be willing to fight for things to happen, even if you are told it can't be done. I have done several things that I was told couldn't be done.

I used the system to give presentations in order to become more visible. When I achieved the MS, my position was perfect for advancement, which was accomplished in a timely fashion. I work in a decentralized, professional-practice model where pure primary nursing is practiced.

Whenever you work within any system, you must agree with the philosophy of that system and feel that you are contributing in a manner worthwhile to the overall functioning as well. I believe that the individual must feel that they are independent and yet a part of the system because there is never going to be a system which completely satisfies the needs of the individual. The system in which I work possesses a very specific mission and works toward the fulfillment of that mission. Overall, the nursing department believes that nursing is a profession, encourages innovative ideas, and is not afraid to take risks. Therefore, an environment is created which allows the individual to work with the system, rather than against the system.

M. Schulte

I have managed the system to my advantage by being assertive and saying what I need and setting my boundaries. I also have learned to play the "game" of politics. I play it well! I feel fine about the game, and accepting it as a part of life makes the challenge fun. Why not enjoy what you have to do!

V. Andrus

I do not think I have managed the system to my advantage. What has helped is for me to learn how *not* to allow the system to manage me. I try to develop one-on-one relationships in the system. I apply Bowen's theory to the work system. That is helpful when I can keep myself out of triangles.

The system in which I work is by most standards a very open system. There is, and has been, increasing encouragement to develop as much as one can within the financial constraints of the institution. Creativity is a key word. Our director of nursing is a very encouraging leader. If we have an idea that we want to try or a system we want to investigate, she encourages us. The system has managed me by encouraging me to stretch and to grow through challenges that I am allowed to seek for myself. I have managed the system by taking those challenges and opportunities when I see them.

J. Sage

The nursing department was my department when I came here. I came as the director of nursing and was made the vice president of nursing. At the current time, we are establishing a totally new delivery-of-care system which maximizes the efforts of the professional nurse.

I have learned to manage the system to my advantage by becoming more politically astute, listening more, observing, discussing, thinking through situations, and mostly by day-to-day experience. The other advantage I have had in the system is my exceptional relationships with physicians over my entire career. I believe my attitude about physicians has not changed dramatically since my original nursing program, and is slightly more positive than what I see in the profession. I was taught to respect and work closely with physicians, and that one could learn from them. I have always held them to a degree of respect and I don't believe ever gave into the current feeling that we must emancipate ourselves by bad-mouthing the medical model. Physicians and nurses are collaborators in the provision of patient care, and this is particularly true in hospitals. I believe that my mutually respectful relationship with physicians has more than paid me back over the years both personally and professionally, and in my ability to run the hospital and problem solve on a day-to-day basis.

From 1979 to the present, I have interfaced with the system (i.e., hospitals and schools of nursing) but have *not* been an employee and will *never* be an employee again!

Since I still practice clinically within the hospital, I'm able to help with nursery staffing, while maintaining my own clinical competence, teach parents, and enjoy patient care. I'm within the system enough to watch it in action, to see the hassles and impossible tasks administration expects of managers and clinical specialists for $30,000 per year! I'm within the system enough to experience its reality. I don't hit myself over the head anymore about going back into the system, that is, being legitimate and having a real job. I don't belong in the system full-time and, if I was there, it would drive me crazy!

S. Gardner

This question is very confusing. I have operated in many systems, that is, organizations, none of which are specifically nursing systems. My 13 years in community mental health exposed me to a multidisciplinary health care system where I functioned as a therapist in many clinical settings. Later, as a generic administrator, I supervised doctors, nurses, social workers, and psychologists. I accessed the system through relationships that I carefully nurtured based on trust and reciprocity. I now work as the only therapist in a medical setting where I must *advocate* for the infertile patient. I also must advocate for therapy as a useful intervention in this high-tech field. I access this system through my same techniques, alliances based on trust and reciprocity.

M. Butterfield

I have managed the system I work in by becoming involved. I like to get a piece of the power and use it. My ideas can't be given a chance if no one hears them. I work in a system of shared governance which allows for these behaviors. However, even in a formerly bureaucratic model, I gained recognition by finding the right channel, working hard, being creative, and joining the right committee.

A. Eckes

Except for one term as a full-time faculty member, my experiences in recent years have been a combination of part-time positions. This has not been accidental. Part-time positions gave me more flexibility in balancing career and family demands. In addition, they allowed me to be a part of a system without some of the extra demands placed on full-time employees, for example, committee appointments and overtime. Recently, I decided to continue my interest in research and computers, and to pursue a management position. I am again combining part-time positions until I find one which combines both interests, or until I can choose one over the other as a primary interest. The disadvantage of managing the system in this way is that one is not part of the day-to-day communication process and, hence, often an outsider, albeit an informed one.

I have had to be more creative as a part-time employee, and that has been stimulating. More than anything else, I've managed the system the way I have to enhance my sense of autonomy. Now that I am further up the ladder, I am examining whether or not I can function happily as an autonomous professional full-time.

E. L. Gallagher

As a vice president and dean, I have a big job! I surround myself with bright, loyal people and delegate. I manage by walking around. I am visible to my constituency and communicate orally and in writing. Positive feedback to my managers is important and so is constructive criticism.

The system I am in is fairly crazy, and I hasten to assure anyone who asks, is probably no crazier than any other system of higher education today, or indeed any business today. I become impatient with people who think nurses are harder on each other than the rest of the world. My own experience has been both in and out of nursing; so I am unable to cherish such delusions. I do not much care for barracudas and nursing has its share. It also has more than its share of dedicated, hard-working, warm people. Academic cannibalism is perhaps more difficult to deal with, since we believed it would not be like the rest of the world. To discover that both academia and health care have become big business is a source of continual frustration. We keep trying to be fair and considerate in a world which is largely shaped by the values of competition, power over, and fear of differences. Obviously we are often caught up in our own hypocrisy, despite our best intentions. We try to be caring at our college, but it gets translated into problems of too many needs, too few resources, and rewards for doing things which may not always be the values shared by nonadministrators. I would not want to be in administration. It seems to me to be a difficult position and one for which others have limited gratitude.

D. Webster

MANAGING THE SYSTEM

Comfort with the workplace was one quality shared by all the successful nurse respondents. These successful nurses occupied just about every role possible, from staff nurse to vice president, from student to professor, and several roles within community nursing. Reading the responses, I would think, "Oh! I could never work there. This person is amazing!" After reacting so to about 90 percent of the responses, I became impressed with the diverse places in which nurses realize success. Apart from comfort with one's workplace, these successful nurses share several other interesting perspectives. They raise issues of "fit" between the person and the work environment; of managing the self versus the system; and of politics.

"Fit" Between the Nurse and the Employing Institution

The "match" between the nurse and the employing institution is called *personal styles analysis* in career-counseling literature. This analysis is a potentially valuable tool for career advancement, if you remember that much of this material is based upon developmental theory and psychological theories that have their roots in Freudian ideas. It is limited in its usefulness to the extent that the male and the pathological base are not generalizable to women who are emotionally healthy. To be fair, the career-counseling literature that I have read in preparing this book is very sensitive to the fact that women are not misshapen men and that neither sex is inherently flawed.

There are several approaches to assessing the fit between self and employing setting. To date, most of these approaches focus on assessing the individual and not the employing setting. So, it would be possible to complete a battery of these tests to determine the best setting for you to flourish in, but you would have little idea of where to find that culture. Adler's individual psychology has been adapted to career decisions by Watkins (1984). The Meyer-Briggs Type Indicator is another popular and useful tool (Keirsey & Bates, 1978; Meyer, 1975, 1980). All of these should be administered by a professional who not only gives the scales, but who uses interviewing skills very well.

In order to go beyond what exists, I shall attempt to address the match between the nurse and the institution, with an emphasis on the institution. Before proceeding though, it will be useful to review some history.

In today's health care environment, it is often difficult to recall that health care, and hospitals in particular, were very unattractive economically until after World War II. Money was lacking; the idea of health insurance was sparked by a teacher's union in Texas and slowly spread. Hospitals were community agencies with little in the way of technology until the Hill-Burton Act was passed after the war. Medical care was as much an art as a science, with few diagnostic procedures and limited therapeutic tools available. Nursing stressed comfort measures, with some teaching when the patient went home. We knew relatively little about nutrition, the pharmacopia was virtually bare, and genetic disorders were viewed with fatalism. Communicable diseases, especially polio, were a major public-health concern.

Tremendous postwar advancements in technology, pharmacology, and most importantly, disease eradication and health promotion as viewed by professionals and the public came with an accompanying sense of optimism. The United States was the first nation in history to successfully deploy arms and simultaneously win on two geographically separate fronts (Germany and Japan). With some justification, we believed we could do anything.

As I reflect upon my own career, the two most influential theories in my life were not developed until after the second World War. They are Rogers' Conceptual Model of Nursing Science and Bowen's Family Systems Theory. Baccalaureate nursing education was also relatively rare. Had I been born 10 years earlier, my life would be totally different!

Hospitals, where most nursing practice and education took place, were much like what Goffman (1961) labeled "asylums" or "total institutions." He defined a total institution as " . . . a place of residence and work where a large number of like-situated individuals, cut off from the wider society for an appreciable period of time, together lead an enclosed, formally administered round of life." This description reflects the 12-hour day, the one-half day off a week, and rules about dress and decorum that typified hospital nursing for years.

All institutions have a tendency to value the ability to become "total" to some extent. The "IBM man" whom one can identify by his white shirt and short haircut is an example of such a tendency. What makes an institution total, however, is that the usual societal pattern wherein one works, sleeps, and plays in different spaces, usually geographically distant from one another and usually involving different persons, is violated. Total-institution reward systems are inner-focused, as opposed to reflecting the values of the larger social system. The idea that one should not be paid for caring, a point of discomfort for nurses, reflects that separation of nursing care from the larger capitalist marketplace. Until recently, under-accounting for revenues and expenditures in the hospital reflected that these institutions were somehow different from others in the society. Granting the technology, therapeutic procedures, and all the rest, the biggest change in hospitals and other health care institutions in the last 40 years is the breakdown of the total institution mentality and the emergence of the capitalist marketplace culture.

The system has turned 180 degrees. Nursing-service departments have changed with it. One of the recurring themes in the comments of the successful nurses is the need to keep current, generally through formal education. As the marketplace becomes the norm in health care, new opportunities open, older career trajectories end, and change is the norm. The current nursing shortage is to a large extent a reflection of the supply-and-demand nature of the American economy. In the past, hospitals had a steady supply of nurses, because as one nurse left to assume family responsibilities, another returned to the workplace. There was a continuous flow. As the health care industry expanded, nurses' options expanded. At the same time, inflation, job loss, and other factors made one income, the male's, insufficient to live on desirably for most families. Now nurses had to work; there were more opportunities and today we have the paradoxical situation whereby more nurses are working than ever before, and yet we still have a nurse shortage. Supply and demand has caught up with nursing.

The same is true for nursing education. Before the women's movement teaching, social work, and nursing were the usual career choices for women. Nursing never had to compete for students. Today, it does. This has led to the creation of nurse-recruiters who use public relations and marketing techniques to attract students.

Given this dynamic state, self- and system-assessment is an important skill to develop. Figure 6.1 presents an assessment model that was developed several years ago at New York University. I find it a bit cumbersome today, but for nurses who have not assessed the fit between themselves and their organization, it is a good exercise.

The column on the left (focal system) is the system you want to understand most clearly. It may be the unit you work on, the entire service, or the whole hospital. The larger the unit of analysis, the more you will have to condense information. For example, in the focal system the objects are the people. If you are examining a nursing unit, you may deal with each individual. If you are assessing the entire institution, you may have to create more general categories, for example, the administration, the nursing-service administration, the nursing staff, the nursing-assistants staff, and so on. You may have to describe their attributes as averages. For example, if you are assessing a nursing unit, you may describe the age, education, sex, race, marital status, and other important variables individually. If you are assessing the nursing-service administration, you may have to describe such variables in aggregates, for example, most are women, their average age, and so on.

The ecological system (center column) is the environment in which the focal system operates. The environment for a nursing unit is the nursing-service department, the entire non-nursing hospital system, and the community. The ecological system for the whole hospital is the community and the state and federal entities that impinge upon its functioning.

The assessor column (right column) refers to you: your goals, values, and so on. The assessment portfolio developed from career-counseling sessions would apply here.

Identification of patterns is the culmination of this exercise. Patterns identify individuals and organizations. They are both hard to change and the only characteristic worth changing to affect the basic organizational culture and methodology.

Finally, you may assess the fit between you and the focal and ecological systems. You need to decide whether that fit is comfortable and workable. For example, you may assess that you are distressed by the "big-business" mentality of the hospital as an ecological system, and its impact on your nursing unit which takes the form of too many patients with too few

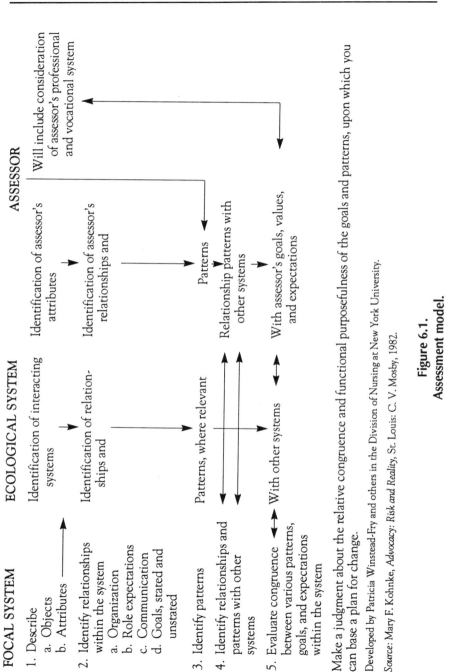

Figure 6.1.
Assessment model.

FOCAL SYSTEM

1. Describe
   a. Objects
   b. Attributes

2. Identify relationships within the system
   a. Organization
   b. Role expectations
   c. Communication
   d. Goals, stated and unstated

3. Identify patterns

4. Identify relationships and patterns with other systems

5. Evaluate congruence between various patterns, goals, and expectations within the system

ECOLOGICAL SYSTEM

Identification of interacting systems

Identification of relationships and

Patterns, where relevant

With other systems

ASSESSOR

Will include consideration of assessor's professional and vocational system

Identification of assessor's attributes

Identification of assessor's relationships and

Patterns

Relationship patterns with other systems

With assessor's goals, values, and expectations

Make a judgment about the relative congruence and functional purposefulness of the goals and patterns, upon which you can base a plan for change.

Developed by Patricia Winstead-Fry and others in the Division of Nursing at New York University.

Source: Mary F. Kohnke, *Advocacy: Risk and Reality,* St. Louis: C. V. Mosby, 1982.

resources. As of 1989, the likelihood that this pattern will change in the foreseeable future is slight. You do not fit. The change will have to come from you. You can become more active politically to try to change the situation. You may move to a less market-oriented hospital (if you can find one). You may become an entrepreneur, consulting on caring and high-quality patient-care maintenance as part of a marketing program for an institution. You may decide to switch careers. You may move to a unit within the organization that is less market-oriented. Whatever option you decide, it will be based upon your assessment of the functional relationship between you and the important systems.

There are nursing models and management approaches that are attractive to nurses. Several of the successful nurses mentioned shared governance, career ladders, primary nursing, patient contracting, and other delivery models as sources of satisfaction. This is not surprising because some of the respondents came from magnet hospitals where these practices are commonplace. The praise of physicians for excellent nursing practice was also mentioned as a source of satisfaction.

This assessment exercise is not designed to induce disappointment or depression. Even if you decide that the focal and ecological systems that surround your work are not what you need and prefer, it is possible to find peace with the inevitable. Victor Frankl (1958) demonstrated that some people, those who found meaning in the suffering, could not only survive the horrors of a Nazi concentration camp, but also grow. If humans can grow under concentration-camp conditions, few can claim that they are totally blocked from career development, even if the setting is less than desirable. This leads to the second theme identified by the successful nurses, managing the self.

Managing the Self versus the System

It is probably clear from the discussions of goal setting, risk taking, and decision making, that one of the secrets of a managed, sensible life is to have a sense of one's self and what one wants. This changes and grows over time, and sometimes becomes complicated, but without it one is buffeted by every wind. A sense of self characterizes all of the successful nurses. Furthermore, one can manage the self by intuition or with logically planned measures.

Any modern health care institution offers outlets for creativity and excellence. Even if informally, one can find satisfaction in mentoring beginning nurses and in providing an excellent role model for students. For some, committee work is a way of moving into powerful positions and for ensuring their voice in management. One way to manage the self was mentioned in avoiding institutional triangles. This idea involves the application of Bowen's Family Systems Theory to organizations.

A triangle is a predictable, automatic response to anxiety. A systems view of the organization requires that one *not* focus on individual personalities, nor on the irritating behavior, nor on the event, but upon the system as a whole. This is not easy because as part of the system, we interact and react with the anxiety. The basic rule for this approach is that the problem resides in the system, not in the individuals.

Triangles become possible because most of us are to some degree emotionally immature and therefore, are not highly functional in all settings. Often we attach emotional needs to our work situation unconsciously. The workaholic is a person who pulls in (triangles in) work to avoid play, family, or whatever his or her unique life problem may be. Workaholics are ultimately detrimental to a system. Good people will leave because the workaholic will not delegate, thus excluding an opportunity to demonstrate their worth and promotability. Similarly, the workaholic often encourages less productive employees to continue in their ways because the workaholic will always be there to pick up the pieces. Workaholism is not the only pattern triangling can take, but it is a common one.

Other people may need to triangle in an issue to decrease the anxiety they experience with a superior. In this case, the triangle looks like Figure 6.2.

The plus sign refers to a feeling of comfort between the two occupants at either end of the line. In this case, the staff-nurse group is comfortable with the dietary department, but the head nurse (the negative line) is embroiled in finding instances of their inefficiency. The relationship between the head nurse and the staff nurses is also comfortable. Comfort in this usage does not mean healthy and functional; it simply means that people are not anxious as long as the triangle stays in place. For example, if the head nurse is embroiled with the deficiencies, real or perceived, of the dietary department, she will not be available to provide leadership in patient care that may be part of her responsibilities.

Triangles are hard to identify because no system is perfect. I used to remind myself when I was in management, that I would not have had a job if organizations could run themselves effectively. What distinguishes a

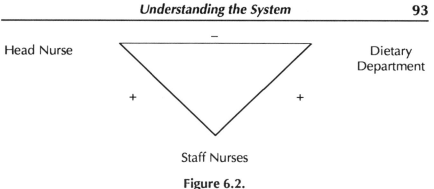

Head Nurse

Dietary
Department

Staff Nurses

Figure 6.2.
Organizational triangle.

triangle from a systems problem is the degree of emotionality surrounding the situation and the fact that such a problem is not solved by reasonable strategies. One of the reasons that hiring people from outside the organization often leads to spectacular success is not only the infusion of "new blood," but because the outsider may break up existing triangles in which they have not become emotionally involved.

Bowen (1978) reports that one of the first clues to anxiety in the system at Georgetown Hospital is that the faculty becomes highly critical of the trainees. In an academic system, it may be one faculty member who is overcriticized, or the students may be perceived as less bright than some previous class. The latter sentiment is fairly easy to tag as a response to anxiety because the odds are minimal that any one faculty member remembers the level of intelligence (whatever that is) for any preceding class.

Anxiety in organizations, as in families, will appear as illness in important persons: conflict; projection onto weaker, less experienced members of the organization. Emotional, physical, or social illness in an important person is an indicator of anxiety in a system. Usually, overtly emotionally ill persons do not advance too far in an organizational hierarchy. However, drug and alcohol abuse and physical illness (ulcers and other so-called psychosomatic illnesses for example) will increase depending upon the level of differentiation of self of the persons involved. [See Bowen (1978), or Miller and Winstead-Fry (1982), for a full description of the concepts in the theory, including differentiation of self. For present reading, consider differentiation of self as equal to emotional maturity.]

Conflict may be overt or covert. In a work setting, conflict between two managers may be particularly unsettling when you are caught in the middle. Dealing with the managers in such a way as not to jeopardize your career requires an understanding of the triangle.

In order to avoid being pulled into triangles, you must be able to take and to maintain an "I position." An I position is a stance that flows from that part of the self that is solid. It is a set of clearly defined opinions, beliefs, and principles that are developed from reflection upon life experiences. These principles are the basis for responsible and informed choices. These principles, opinions, and beliefs can be maintained in high-anxiety situations. In contrast to these beliefs and principles are those developed by the pseudo-self. The pseudo-self is that portion of the self that appears solid until anxiety builds up. The beliefs, opinions, and principles that reside here can be abandoned, like a ship, when the emotional winds are too stormy. Each of us has probably had an experience with someone whom we thought "really had it together," and then changed completely when some issue produced a high level of anxiety.

An I position is not a defensive position. It is the simple, clear assertion of where one stands without denigrating or diminishing where others stand. Suppose, for example, the head nurse cited earlier tries to enlist the help of a staff nurse in dealing with the deficiencies of the dietary department. Suppose also, that the staff nurse assessed that the situation was a triangle. The staff nurse's involvement would entail hours of emotional discussion about how bad the dietary department was (perhaps invading her personal time), writing memos, and documenting events of dubious importance. An I statement in this situation may sound something like, "Mary Ann (head nurse's name), I am all for providing the best patient care, but my priorities are such that the dietary department is low on the list." It may take persistence to dissuade Mary Ann, but the I position allows the staff nurse to avoid the emotionality of Mary Ann's cause. Usually, if the situation is really a triangle, if one does not feed into the emotionality, the person (head nurse Mary Ann) will retreat fairly soon.

Politics

Successful nurses understand that politics exist, and they can play the game if they so desire. Talbott and Vance (1981) define politics as "influencing the allocation of scarce resources." Mason and Talbott

(1985) point out that only recently has politics become a part of nursing curriculum, nursing practice discussions, and research. They suggest that "nice girls don't do that" (p. 4) because the word *politics* conjures images of double dealing and smoked-filled rooms. My interpretation would be that Mason is correct, and the tendency to avoid politics was reinforced because of the total-institution situation that characterized nursing training and practice when the hospital was the primary setting for both. As Goffman (1961) points out, rules are so prescribed and so inculcated in total institutions that any notion that they might be negotiated, a basic political skill, is never even considered; so political skills are not developed.

The other barrier to the development of political skills is the historic lack of team sports in women's formative years. Team sports teach us how to accomplish goals with people even if you do not like them. For example, if you want to play baseball, you need nine team members. That is a game rule. You need to convince nine people that they would rather be playing ball than watching television, or whatever. It is inevitable that some of these people are going to be unliked. The situation is even more dramatic if you need a good shortstop, and you have to ask someone you dislike to play for the good of the team. Henning and Jardim (1977), in their classic study of women managers, report that creating a team based upon competence and not personal preference was a skill their successful businesswomen had to learn.

A doctoral student who was interviewing deans for her dissertation interviewed me. Part of the interview had to do with childhood and skills learned then that are useful in current activities. I was recounting my lifelong love of baseball and expertise in high school as a guard in basketball. She was surprised that I valued this so much. I asked her to include a question about sports in the future and to go back to previous interviewees and ask them about this. It was interesting that *all* of us either played team sports as children, were "tomboys," or made a conscious effort to learn the skills of team membership and negotiating that come naturally from this activity. Several of the deans credited spouses or mentors with specifically teaching them how to go about building an effective team and how to overcome personal dislikes and focus on competencies needed to pursue goals.

Some degree of political sophistication is needed to navigate through life. Increasingly, nursing education is including political issues and skills. Nursing organizations are including workshops on political skills in meetings and in materials distributed to members. Nursing political actions coalitions are viewed as quite effective by elected officials. The nurses' lobby in Washington is a real force in that arena.

The system, in whatever form it takes, is a real force for happiness, success, defeat, or stagnation in one's career. Leadership in managing the system/organization comes from all places in the hierarchy. In decentralized models, for a nurse to be perceived as effective, she must interact in a proactive manner. In this model, not to participate is equivalent to sabotaging the organization. In hierarchical systems, it may require moving up the hierarchical ladder to have impact; committees may provide the avenue; or succeeding the conventional wisdom that says "it cannot be done" may be the road to establishing a powerful voice. Whatever the organizational setting and wherever one's position within it, organizational/system issues will impinge and shape one's practice and opportunities for development and advancement in some ways. To progress within an organization, effective methods for dealing with these issues proactively must be developed.

7

Family and Personal Characteristics

I am the third of four children, an only daughter. My father was American and died of cancer when I was five. Among my memories of him is a visit from the VSN and seeing his colostomy stoma. My mother, an Irish immigrant, was 40 when my father died and my brothers were 8, 7, and almost 3 years. My mothers was a hard worker and a good manager, so my childhood was happy. She says she involved us in her decision making because she had no one else to talk things over with. One of her sisters always lived with us, and another was with us for a few years. We also had a young woman who roomed with us for a few years. We lived in a four-room apartment with one bathroom, so cooperation was required and not discussed.

While my mother valued education highly, it came first for the sons. They were to be catered to and waited on and not expected to do any household chores. They were expected to contribute money from their paper routes to the household and the older boys had routes at age eight. While I was loved, I was aware at an early age of the double standard for males and females, and the value that was attached to "real" work and the income it generated.

My first job was in a five-and-dime store when I was 16. I worked 25 hours per week. I always was drawn to health care, except for a brief time when I thought about majoring in math. Early in high school I thought about being a doctor and decided that was impractical financially and because I wanted to marry and have a large family. Retrospectively, I would not have had the grades either. Fortunately, I went to a high school which prepared me for one thing: to go to college. When my mother suggested it was time for me to get a job, preferably with the telephone company, or that I go to a diploma school if I was going to be a nurse. I firmly fought for what I wanted and went to college. I've always been an achiever. In my very early years, I did well because of my ability, and later I was further fueled by wanting to prove girls were not only as good as, but better than boys! I'm sure that nursing appealed to me because I thought it was mostly women and that they were running their own show.

I am the first-born girl [in my family]. My younger sister died at birth and so I am an only child (more like the oldest child-type of only children). Mom was born in Japan and left a tiny village after World War II to go to cooking and sewing school in Tokyo. There she met my dad, a white, American Army officer, and they married.

My mother is really intelligent, but post-secondary school wasn't possible for any but the most elite women in those days. After several years on an Army base in Okinawa, I grew up in Phoenix in an ultra-conservative, white, suburban neighborhood. When dad retired from the Army, he said that either he or she should be the home person. Mom stayed home because they thought he had the greater earning potential. Mom stayed home with me until I started high school. I think she was much happier once she started working outside the home. Neither of my parents followed a formal religion, although they did provide the opportunity for me to do so, which I did for 10 years. I don't consider myself a Methodist or a Christian, but I was very enriched by my experience with the Methodist Church. My dad was very involved in affirmative action at his work. I was very involved with academic and extracurricular activities in grade- and high school. I was a Girl Scout through my first year of college, and this was a major influence. I was constantly exposed to capable, intelligent, caring women (and men). The Scouts really opened my eyes to the value of supporting and helping others and to the range of possibilities for women. I've often been a little surprised that I became a nurse. My dad was proud; my mom was really upset.

I am the first born. I have one sister two and one-half years younger. My parents were both alcoholics. My father died of liver disease (due to alcohol). My mother was left with a six-year-old and an eight-year-old. She drank herself into oblivion and I literally raised my sister. I cleaned and cooked and cared for their needs. Often I would return from school and she was so drunk I couldn't awaken her. Thus, I am the typical child of an alcoholic. I attempt to be everything to everyone, often putting my own self in jeopardy.

I grew up in a very strict, traditional, Catholic family. I also went to parochial schools. Therefore, I believe the concept of angel of mercy; helping others, taking care of others, giving of yourself was strongly reinforced. It seemed the two choices for women were teacher or nurse. I received very much support from family, teachers, friends, and parents to become an RN. I was the second child of four girls. I basically had many caretaker responsibilities: raising my two younger sisters, household chores, groceries, cooking, cleaning. We lived on a farm so we all had to work together.

I grew up in a family with a dominating mother who controlled my every move and a father who was mostly absent even when he was physically present. My mother used me as a confidante since I was a teenager and showed her love conditionally. I think part of my going into nursing came from the familial responsibility of caretaking for my mother and from my wanting to get attention for being a good and helpful person. I do not see these as positive reasons for becoming a nurse and have, for several years, been working at not being a caretaker for everyone with the motive of getting attention and appreciation. As I learn to love myself more, I need to get recognition less and less from outside myself. A disconnection with my family has been a sad yet freeing part of my life.

My mother is a homemaker; my father is a businessman. Both are first-generation Americans who are well accomplished, well educated, and socially involved. They have worked hard and sacrificed for their children to make a better life, to assimilate into the mainstream culture through education and drive. They are not nurturing people, however. They also have very high expectations of their children with little psychological insight into their own behavior. My siblings were relatively isolated from myself and each other due to four- and five-year age differences. My family never dealt well with conflict. Both of my parents have a lot of unexpressed rage which tended to escape at frequent intervals with petty quarreling and yelling. I'm sure nursing has been a way for me to develop that nurturing part of myself, a self-healing, and perhaps a counterdependency in that caring for others enhances my self-esteem. There is a balancing act to guard against using caring for others as a way to avoid dealing with my own needs. There is a security in nursing, knowing that financially there will always be a way to make a living.

I grew up in a loving, stable family in suburban New Jersey. Both parents are in the health profession. I think there was a natural tendency for me to choose nursing, although my only sibling did not choose a health-related career.

Neither of my parents were college graduates, but they had a sense of stability, ethics, and love. I learned very young that to always be who you were was most important. My father always tried to be who he wasn't and had many personal failures. My mother was true to herself and has a strength and wisdom about her. I was the oldest of two [children]. The second is a brother who never completed college. He lives in a rural area, a very simple, nonmaterial life, with his wife and two children. He is very fundamental in his religious beliefs and sees mainly black and white. We are very different in perspective, but very close because of an acceptance of each other's ways. My parents have never really understood me because of my "untraditional ways," but I have always felt loved and respected. My successes have always surprised them in some ways because they did not see me seeking them.

Like many women who become nurses, I'm from a dysfunctional family. I had a physically violent, alcoholic father and a passive-aggressive, dependent mother. As the oldest child/female, I assumed the role of mother to my brothers, sisters, and mother at nine years of age. Unlike the rest of the family, I wouldn't "keep the family secret" of alcoholism. I confronted my mother, father, relatives, adult friends, clergy, lawyers, and called it what it was. My father is also a domineering, Southern male who was adamant against me going to Catholic high school and becoming a nurse. I was supposed to do whatever it was he wanted me to do (just like my battered mother), but of course I wasn't to know what that was (or what the consequences would be for not complying). I had to make a decision to be whatever he wanted me to be (the hidden agenda, i.e., complete control) or do what I wanted to do. I also had to figure out what the consequences would be: losing love, losing financial and emotional support—great decision for a 12-year-old. I made the right decision, to be true to myself! I've lived with the consequences of that choice; I've supported and educated myself since I was 12 years old. I learned very early to deal with reality, not what I'd like the situation to be, or I wouldn't survive. As one of my therapists stated, "You have a perfect right to be psychotic." I believe in what Peck states in *The Road Less Traveled*, that mental health is an "ongoing process of dedication to reality at all costs."

My early life taught me many lessons: (1) assess the *reality* of the situation; (2) assess risk/benefit of the situation; (3) assess the "price" of compliance/non-compliance; (4) in the end, be true to yourself! In the end, we are in control only of, and are responsible only for ourselves, our choices, and our behavior.

FAMILY OF ORIGIN INFLUENCES

No names were cited with the family descriptions because I did not have, nor did I want to obtain the consent of family members to publish their names. The successful nurses overwhelmingly came from functional families. Nurses who achieved success, who came from unhappy backgrounds were the minority, comprising not more than 12 percent of the group. The nurse who states, "like many women who become nurses, I'm from a dysfunctional family," is either wrong, over-generalizing, or not referring to successful nurses.

The relationship of childhood experiences to adult life, while theoretically postulated, is not well documented from a research perspective. How childhood relates to later career success is even less empirically studied. There are few longitudinal studies of childhood to adulthood. Probably the most successful such study is Terman's study of geniuses who indeed do better in adult life: They have happy marriages, do well economically, and perceive their lives as meaningful.

Erikson, Erikson, and Kivnick (1986), in *Vital Involvement in Old Age*, interviewed 29 persons who were picked up between January 1, 1928 and June 30, 1929 at the Institute of Child Welfare in Berkeley, California. The people were part of the Guidance Study, one of three longitudinal studies begun in 1927. The participants were children of professors and others associated with the University of California, so this was by no means a random sample. However, a remarkable amount of data was compiled on these people. In 1960 the institute offered to make the materials available to selected researchers. The data for the early years is remarkably complete, assembled from regular home visits to the families until the children were 16 years old.

Erikson, Erikson, and Kivnick interviewed these 29 persons in detail, based upon Erikson's stages of development. They focused upon the later stages of development, generativity, and integrity, because that was their interest and that was the age of the sample. These participants were children during the Depression, very often soldiers during World War II, and the parents of the "baby-boom" generation. Their study did not focus on career success, although from the descriptions of their homes and from their comments, most of the persons were living decently, if not comfortably.

Generally, participants experienced ups and downs over the life cycle. Some were characterized as having more dystonic tendencies than strengths which were painful. However, the authors state,

> At this point, we must emphasize that, regardless of what may appear to be individual success or failure in re-experiencing the psychosocial themes of a life-time, our elders are all involved in the process of trying. It is this effort that is the basis for growth at all stages of the life cycle. (pp. 72–73)

Most of the participants had maintained contact with children and grandchildren. A few were disappointed that the "perfect" child was an unemployed, sort of lost adult who never succeeded. The stories of the participants, however, suggest that their children were generally doing well financially, emotionally, and parentally. The study did not attempt to distinguish successful male and female children. This is not meant as a criticism of the study, but it does limit the study's usefulness to the present discussion of families with children who go on to become successful nurses, most of whom are women.

The material in the Erikson, Erikson, and Kivnick interviews parallels the findings of Belenky, Clinchy, Goldberger, and Tarule (1986) mentioned earlier. Women who achieved more autonomous epistemological levels had "good enough" parents and teachers. These adults were not always the most supportive or emotionally available, especially fathers; they did not denigrate the daughters; most encouraged educational pursuits; and they listened often enough and well enough for these young women to feel that they were being heard by their parents.

Belenky and her co-authors also showed that parental-interaction patterns changed over the life cycle. Fathers became more nurturing and emotionally aware as they aged (perhaps akin to Erikson's ideas of intimacy and generativity). Mothers, often silent in their early years, became more active and self-sufficient as they matured. Other research has also suggested that over time, parents and children do grow and change in ways that are mutually supportive (Neugarten, 1969; Rossi, 1980).

While one certainly wishes that every child would have a happy childhood—and from the comments of the successful nurses, most did— a happy childhood does not seem to predict success. Indeed Belenky and her colleagues found incidences of incest and abuse beyond those generally reported in a standard psychiatric textbook (1986, p. 59), and some of the successful women entrepreneurs Jennings (1987) studied also reported rough times in childhood.

If one wants to pursue familial influences in their current life, the genogram introduced in Chapter 2 may be useful to trace patterns across generations, with an emphasis on dysfunctional families. To gain more understanding of how to use the genogram for this purpose, refer to Guerin and Pendagast (1976) or to Miller and Winstead-Fry (1982); both sources are listed in the References.

NUCLEAR FAMILIES/CURRENT FAMILY

The personal strengths that I possess are that I am a mover and a shaker, and that I obtain my goals. My major weakness is that I take on too many things and sometimes I find myself overwhelmed. However, I am committed to meeting deadlines, and usually do. I grapple with the fact that I work long hours (50–60 hours a week) and I do not spend enough time with my family. However, my husband is very supportive of my career choice and he has taken a more complete role within our family. We share both family and home responsibilities and do not "keep count." If I cannot do something, then he will, and I know I can count on him.

. . . . Nor am I willing to place my family and my career in opposing corners.

(This successful nurse made this comment in the context of discussing risks that are unacceptable.)

In the last five years, I really have recommited myself to nursing, and have become more involved in continuing education (in graduate school), professional organizations, and nursing committees at my place of employment. My children are older and more independent, and I have more time to devote to my own career.

My best decision is never to let my career be an excuse for poor mothering or poor spouse relationships, and vice versa.

How do you live the balance of career and family? And caring about self? This is a difficult challenge. At times it overwhelms me. It is unlikely to become easier in the future. I do not get to devote as much time to my daughters as I would like. I fear they are growing up quickly without me. They are three and six years old. I cannot say no to a new research and practice project without abandoning aspects of my dream. I feel a commitment to further publications, so that others will share my vision of what nursing can be, and so that the focus of health care in this society will slowly change in accordance with my dream. There is not enough time, and I do not have enough strength to do it all well, consistently. Also, I am committed to caring about self, which I live primarily through exercise. I rapidly deviate from who I want to be when I put off exercise for more than 48 hours. I need to exercise as an important way of caring about myself. Balancing all of these promises to self and others is my major struggle in being the nurse I am. It calls for all of my creativity and places demands on those I love most, no matter how I choose. I strongly suggest that other happy nurses share this struggle.

I believe it is very hard to balance career and personal life, at least I have found that to be one of the greatest challenges given that a career requires so much time and energy, as well as commitment to carry it through. Although I do believe that it is possible to achieve a balance, I do think that it is very difficult in the present climate and the social change process that is going on in our society to achieve a balance that is seen by all key players in one's personal and professional field as positive and workable.

These comments sound like those of all working women. For those of us who try to challenge stereotypes, the fifth response is from a male nurse. The challenges of balancing career and family are big issues for many women today. There are multiple programs and books dealing with this challenge, and to my knowledge, no one has found the one correct formula. I think the respondent who commented that she never accepts career as an excuse for family, and vice versa, has raised an interesting point, because it reflects my own experience.

The underlying assumption in the idea of balance between career and family is that both entities are dichotomous and that this is a new phenomenon. I can honestly say that I have never had to make an either/or decision, for several reasons:

1. I do not buy into the dichotomous view. From my reading of history, women have always been extraordinarily busy. I cannot believe that the pioneer women of the 19th century, who were responsible for gardening, clothes making, child rearing, and canning food and

curing meat were any less busy than I am. Life is a challenge and sometimes rough, but there is a flow of responsibility and continuity that women have experienced historically. I think a follower of Jung could probably even find me an archetype to express this idea better.

2. We have one child. That does limit the developmental stages one is dealing with simultaneously. However, because I believe that only children need exposure to other children and families, I spend a lot of time picking up and delivering assorted children.

3. When my daughter was in elementary school, I worked across the street from my home. This was a mixed blessing. Every now and then she would run across the street toward the university without looking and it seemed as though every employee of the New York University campus security would call to tell me about the incident. I could spend a lot of time on the phone!

4. I was very successful with babysitters. (I will discuss babysitters further.)

5. We had enough money and lived in New York City. I could usually find a way around a problem. Once I hired a licensed practical nurse to care for our daughter and her babysitter, both sick with miserable colds, because I had to attend a budget meeting. The nurse was not pleased with my use of her skills, but everyone made it to work and our babysitter and our daughter had a good day.

6. My husband and I have a good business relationship. We get done what needs to get done. I think that is what the successful nurse was referring to when she said she and her husband share chores and "don't count." Furthermore, getting done what needs to be accomplished can often be funny. I received my first invitation to publish a paper when our daughter was about one year of age. She was half crawling and half walking, and was into everything. I think she could move at the speed of light. I had one weekend to get the paper done, and we had a party to go to on Saturday night. There was no time to lose, and the heat was off in my office to accommodate a boiler repair. I took the typewriter into the bathroom, placed it on the toilet seat, curled up in lotus position, and started typing. This was fine, until the dog gave my hiding place away! Finally, my husband and daughter went to the park until I had a draft. It also pays to be an excellent typist.

I certainly would not recommend my approach to everyone. If there is truth to the idea that to some extent we create our reality by our belief system, whether one believes one is dealing with a dichotomy or whether one doesn't see dichotomies, will offer different options for actions.

Baby Sitters

Along with microwave ovens and crock pots, the babysitter is likewise an indispensable tool for the working mother. My family always comments that I and one other cousin (also a nurse) never seem to have the babysitter troubles that plague others. In comparing notes with my cousin, we developed a few ideas that I pass on for what they are worth:

1. There are cultural differences in how mothers hold their young, cuddle them, talk to them, and so on. It was important for me to have a babysitter who was a member of my culture. Living in New York City at that time, I advertised in a local ethnic newspaper and received 12 responses.

2. Babysitters serve two functions: (1) They take care of the baby; and (2) they contribute to the smooth functioning of the household. A babysitter who is constantly sick or late, although great with the children, is not fulfilling his or her functions.

3. When I interviewed potential babysitters, all of whom were quite acceptable, I had them spend some time with the baby, holding the baby and doing whatever seemed natural to the potential babysitter. I selected the babysitter who made me the most jealous of the relationship I could envision her developing with our baby. (My husband also liked her the best.)

4. The relationship between babysitter and child is a separate relationship with its own pattern. Once we were satisfied that the babysitter was competent, we stayed out of the relationship. In our case, the babysitter was much younger than we were. Indeed she was at a more appropriate age to be having a first child than we were! She and our daughter walked and ran and shared a very high-energy time. This was nice because the baby would go to bed and would sleep all night.

5. Children will get mad and be dreadful whether the mother works or

not. Terrible two's are terrible and they know how to hurt! I can remember the first time my daughter told me she loved her babysitter more than me. After the initial "ouch," I congratulated myself on the fine job I did of picking our babysitter. I do not think one should hire babysitters who make you uncomfortable, and once hired, periodic evaluations of how things are going are in order. However, I have seen mothers who get so jealous of the fine relationship between their child and the sitter that they find a reason to fire him or her. By determining at the start that the babysitter-child relationship is separate, and not a substitute for a mother-child relationship, some emotional turmoil can be avoided.

6. I never had the babysitter perform housework because it is easier to evaluate if the bathroom has been cleaned than it is to evaluate if the child was hugged. I also must comment that our sitter would do the wash and some cleaning spontaneously, if the baby slept for a long time. I always paid her additionally for this.

7. I always paid babysitters, usually teenagers, who do the occasional evening or Saturday at least half of what they would have made if I cancelled. This practice probably accounts for the fact that my cousin and I can always get a sitter. We never leave them without some income that they might have been counting on, and they express their appreciation by being available. For me, this was also a feminist issue, for a woman's time is always valuable, not just when someone with power wants to pay for it. I am amused that several of my former sitters have gone into business and have had no trouble charging reasonable fees for their services. I hope I contributed to that.

I am not sure everyone could follow my path in dealing with babysitters, but it was successful for my family. Our daughter had the same sitter for the first five years of her life, and they got together a couple of times a year for a period after that. As our daughter approached five and a full-day kindergarten experience became available, we worked out a schedule so the sitter could go to secretarial school, which was her goal.

We certainly strained the budget to have the continuity in babysitting that we enjoyed. It is a temporary situation, and the sense of security that came from having the same people most of the time was worth it.

PERSONALITY CHARACTERISTICS

I am creative, strong, innovative, risk-taking, passionate, person-oriented, nonsexist, masculine, and hedonic. I am also obtuse, weak, fearful, and uncertain. It does not make much sense to me to label any of these as strengths or weaknesses. The most important things to me are being affiliative with others, and being open to joy. My images of self change constantly as I struggle in the yesterday and tomorrow of the now. Another important aspect of self, for me, is my valuing of colleagues. For example, it is of extreme personal importance to me that I drop *everything* when a student asks for guidance or help. It is important to me that I help that person as I myself have been helped by others. Knowing who I am, I move beyond my present images of self toward new pictures of myself together with others. Painful struggle, to be sure. And it brings me to the only joy I can find.

I like to create new programs and be out there giving them away. I really enjoy empowering others. I get excited when I see another person sparked by enthusiasm because we have interacted. I think one of my strengths is I don't revere anyone. I do have great respect for some people though. However, we all came in and will go out the same way; so we can all contribute as we are given the chance and/or take it. I don't mind hard work, however, I will not do it just for the sake of doing it. I think I developed all my strengths as I went along. I used to be so afraid of people, and I have worked very hard to overcome fear. I still feel it sometimes, but refuse to let it get in my way. I have some incredible people in my life that support me in moving on and growing. These relationships continue to develop. I feel it is vital to find people that will provide lasting, open, honest relationships both as mentors and counselors, and as friends and supporters. I have been lucky (actually I worked at that too; so it wasn't luck) to find some very special people.

A weakness that I grapple with is that I sometimes just want to do nothing which makes it difficult to think about moving ahead again. Another weakness/limitation is that I *hate* doing research and I have to do it to evaluate my program effectively. Lastly, I am sometimes too lenient or caring when what a person really needs a good kick in the pants. (That probably comes from a fear of rejection, and I am definitely working on it.)

I believe that one of the greatest personal strengths that I have, and which I think can be generalized to leaders, is the ability to interact well with people and to assess the strengths and weaknesses of others rather rapidly. I enjoy being friendly, outgoing, and interactive with not only members of my own professional discipline, but with those of other groups as well. I enjoy projects that are interdisciplinary and bridge the "bigger issue" problems. I also like to see a project completed and therefore will persevere until I have achieved my given goal and objective, rather than to start and not finish most projects. I believe that good interpersonal communication is generally a natural part of my personality, but there is no doubt that the combination of formal education and learning on the job has enhanced and assisted me in developing this skill further.

I believe that taking on too many projects is definitely a problem. It is difficult, given many opportunities, to be selective and start to weed out those projects which are less interesting or which will yield less than exciting outcomes. Therefore, I think that I am grappling with the need to be more selective in what projects I take on.

N. Valentine

My personal strengths, in my opinion are assertiveness, sensitivity, a drive for knowledge, and a lean toward perfectionism which helps me push others to do their best. Some of these strengths are a very natural part of my personality and others were parts that may have been there all along, but had to be more finely tuned.

Weaknesses? Limitations? This is, of course, a very hard thing to admit when there is a tendency toward perfectionism! Sometimes I can feel a strength becoming a limitation, especially when dealing with others. It is very hard not to expect the same strength from them. I also have a tendency toward impatience. I want things done yesterday! This is possibly the most difficult to deal with, as I cannot accomplish the things I want to in the time I'd like to do it in.

J. Sage

My personal strengths and weaknesses were developed as survival strategies in childhood. I am decisive, independent, and assertive. I believe that nothing is impossible, that I can do anything I set my mind to. I am confident of my own personal power. I'm definitely a leader, not a follower; I'm creative and a problem solver, and love the challenge of an adventure, a risky proposition. I'm direct, straightforward, and confronting; I don't manipulate. I have high moral and ethical standards, both personally and professionally. I value integrity, sincerity, and honesty. I'm a hard worker and hard-playing, after learning to relax as an adult! I'm an advocate for babies, children, and families.

The "flipside" of my strengths are my weaknesses. I can be tactless, impatient . . . intolerant, unforgiving and unforgetting, blunt, angry, and overpowering/intimidating.

As I've become older, I have attempted to temper these negative aspects of my strengths. I've also "mellowed with age." I'm choosier about the windmills I tilt. I am clearer about what I want and don't want; what I'll tolerate/negotiate and what is untenable and non-negotiable. I don't waste my time, energy, and life on the latter.

Sandy Gardener

PERSONAL CHARACTERISTICS

The comments offered by the successful nurses read like those of successful women in any occupation: there is no one "success" personality, but rather a general sense of being able to manage life and to continue to grow. Jennings, in discussing women entrepreneurs interviewed for her book, *Self-Made Women,* comments:

> They are possessed of tremendous self-confidence, an energy and willingness to work hard, and a strong sense of femininity that they are unwilling to sacrifice. In addition, they show an increasing resistance to the idea of having to choose between career and home in order to succeed. (p. 24)

Rather than a self-assessment exercise, I offer the following exercise, "Guess Who's Being Quoted." The quotes are either from successful nurses, successful women who are not nurses, or nurse entrepreneurs. My hunch is that the reader will not be able to identify one from the other consistently.

Guess Who's Being Quoted

Based on the statements given, select the individual you believe was most likely to have made the statement:

1. My basic mistake—where all my other mistakes came from—was underestimating my own strength; always thinking that there was someone else who knew more or could do it better than I.

   _____ Successful nurse

_____ Nurse entrepreneur

_____ Successful woman, non-nurse

2. I mapped out this ideal job two years ago; my list had about 20 requirements. Every requirement was met, except that I'm earning more money than anticipated. I love all aspects of what I'm doing. I can be all I want to be.

_____ Successful nurse

_____ Nurse entrepreneur

_____ Successful woman, non-nurse

3. I could not achieve my goals without being assertive. I think that even years ago, when the word *assertive* was not such a popular word for women, I was still being assertive in order to get/be what I envisioned for myself.

_____ Successful nurse

_____ Nurse entrepreneur

_____ Successful woman, non-nurse

4. I learned to hire people with skills different than mine, to appreciate other ways of working in order to complement my style, and to delegate (most difficult).

_____ Successful nurse

_____ Nurse entrepreneur

_____ Successful woman, non-nurse

5. Yes, I made the mistake of not charging enough. I had no idea what the going rate was. I didn't know anyone else who was doing what I was doing so I couldn't even compare rates.

_____ Successful nurse

_____ Nurse entrepreneur

_____ Successful woman, non-nurse

6. Even if you don't want it to happen, business and personal lives are liable to seep into each other. At home I can become preoccupied

with what's happening with work. And while I'm here, I worry about home.

_____ Successful nurse

_____ Nurse entrepreneur

_____ Successful woman, non-nurse

7. A willingness to take risks, determination, and a blind passion for what I do are the strengths that I bring to the business and its growth.

_____ Successful nurse

_____ Nurse entrepreneur

_____ Successful woman, non-nurse

8. I have abundant energy, a positive attitude, drive, organization skills, and salesmanship. These are the strengths I bring to my business, which provides in-service education services, program design and evaluation, meeting management, legal consultation, and promotions and marketing to a variety of institutions.

_____ Successful nurse

_____ Nurse entrepreneur

_____ Successful woman, non-nurse

9. I am most of all a survivor. That is my greatest strength. My greatest weakness is also a strength (every other day) and that is a need to try to make sense of things that probably don't make sense.

_____ Successful nurse

_____ Nurse entrepreneur

_____ Successful woman, non-nurse

10. Women are seen as givers. And when you are doing something that involves women, it is assumed that you will give, give, give. Now, I'm finally learning to say no, but it's still difficult for me.

_____ Successful nurse

_____ Nurse entrepreneur

_____ Successful woman, non-nurse

The answers to this exercise are

1. A successful woman, non-nurse, discussing her shoe-importing business, in response to a question about mistakes she made.

2. A nurse entrepreneur discussing the self-confidence she brings to her work.

3. One of the successful nurses in commenting upon the role of assertiveness in pursuing her goals.

4. A nurse entrepreneur discussing the interpersonal skills that are needed to succeed.

5. A successful woman, non-nurse, discussing mistakes she made in building up her picture-research business.

6. A successful woman, non-nurse, discussing advice she would give women interested in starting a business.

7. A nurse entrepreneur discussing the growth of her business.

8. A nurse entrepreneur discussing the physical and mental resilience required to set up a business.

9. One of the successful nurses commenting upon her decision-making style.

10. A successful woman, non-nurse, discussing the problems of making money in a business that services women.

All of the quotes from nurse entrepreneurs were taken from Vogel and Doleysh, *Entrepreneuring: A Nurse's Guide to Starting a Business*, pages 28, 29, 26, 31. The quotes of successful women, non-nurses, were taken from Moran's *Invest in Yourself: A Woman's Guide to Starting Her Own Business*, pages 138, 141, 155, 175. The successful nurses' comments come from my interviews.

The idea that there is a constellation of personality characteristics that lead to success in nursing is intriguing, but does not predict the success of a nurse. Whatever the sources of success, women who achieve success are themselves, varied individuals, who share a common denominator that is the drive and commitment that are needed to do anything well.

8

Mentors

Several people have influenced my career development, two of whom I consider mentors. Both of these people are educators, doctorally-prepared nurses, women, and mothers. One mentor was a teacher in my master's program; the other was a teacher in my doctoral program. Each person, at the time, presented a role model for the next step in my career. Each of these women encouraged my development, professionally and personally. They supported and shaped critical-thinking skills, wrote letters of support when I was ready to move on, provided invaluable advice when asked, and introduced me to a wider network of nurses than I had been exposed to previously. The negative effects were negligible in comparison to the benefits.

Very young in my career, I took a risk in reporting behavior by my head nurse that I deemed unsafe to patients. I was removed from the specific unit, but was retained by the hospital. For eight years following that, I took no risks. Under a wonderful mentor, in the last two years, I have taken some risks. For example, I developed a proposal for an education center for the community providing a diversity of services from prenatal education to stop-smoking classes. I have nurses marketing hospital services to attending physicians. Staff nurses decide on the final hires for their units.

No mentors have been part of my career advancement.

K. Barry-Bellis

My mentor was a professor at the University of Arizona. She encouraged me to grow and develop in my career. I moved from hospital nursing to nurse-case management after 17 years in nursing. It's not easy to change jobs after 20 years in one institution.

I hate this question! So many people helped and inspired me, but I can't say who has been my mentor! I owe a lot to Jin Chin, the head nurse at my first job; to Mary Henrikson, a colleague who pushes me and gives me ground-breaking opportunities like important speaking engagements; and to Pam Jordan, PhD, a faculty member who encouraged me to start my private practice and thinks I'm wonderful.

The only negative aspects of mentors is when you want someone to be your mentor and they don't! Some people I greatly admire have ignored me.

G. Wall

I had a nurse-political mentor beginning in 1983. She encouraged me and taught me. She also supported me in everything I tried, allowing me to learn through many of my own failures as I grew. No negative aspects. She is still available and friendly and supportive. We share more than mentoring now, but she still listens and encourages and debates with me.

I have had three mentors! First was a staff nurse who taught me to be a nurse when I was a student extern working at a hospital between my junior and senior years of college. I still say she made me a nurse! My second mentor was in my master's program. She was my nursing theory professor who guided my thesis research and taught me to trust my abilities to do research. My third mentor was a teacher in my certificate program in nurse midwifery. At that time, she was finishing her dissertation. She heartily encouraged me to pursue a doctorate. We used to get together to just "talk research." She is still my source of intellectual stimulation and encouragement. I haven't had negative experiences in my experiences with these mentors.

My pediatric instructor was my first mentor. I am sure that is the reason I first pursued that area. The vice president of nursing where I work was my mentor for the past four years. She had great faith in me and frequently recommended me for projects, committees, and honors. We shared ideas and dreams about nursing together. One dream is now becoming a reality. Bedside computers are being installed. The only negative aspect I can think of is that your association or close tie with someone may not be liked by others.

E. Godfrey

The only mentor I can say I had was my aunt who inspired me to become a nurse and guided me to the BSN program. Beyond that, I have been on my own, inspired by my father's words to get some education and do something with my life.

D. Quinn

There have been several mentors, but one in particular was Marilyn Pires, the rehabilitation clinical specialist at University Hospital in Boston. She inspired me to search out and seek professional avenues which otherwise I might not have known about or would have taken a lot longer to discover.

M. Finnell

I have not had any mentors, per se, but several nurses have been role models: D. Del Bueno, J. Fawcett, and two work colleagues. One nurse is a woman whom I admired as a student nurse, and to this day she remains an outstanding professional leader.

J. Pond

My first mentor was my now brother-in-law. He was the first person I knew who had a professional career. I was eight or so; he believed in me, and told me I could do anything I wanted to. It stuck! In my first two nursing positions, I had very strong nursing supervisors. I really admired and looked up to them. They responded to me as if they saw something special in me. They challenged me to reach beyond that which I thought I was capable of. These were not close or long relationships, but that ability to give the challenge and to step back and be in the wings saying we know that you can do this is still very vivid. There have been no other mentors. I've come to think of myself as being a "hardy personality" and "self sufficient." The negative is it's occasionally lonely.

M. Sprik

I worked for a woman through the first nine years in my positions in this organization. Through that time, she offered a lot of developmental opportunities; [she] supported my growth, and promoted me into higher level management positions. I respected her achievements and her professionalism. I used her as a role model. We did not have close, intimate discussions about my career, nor did she step out of her role as my supervisor in guiding my pathway. I have played mentor to many women in the organization by being available to share views and experiences where relevant. I have given advice when asked and discussed the political climate to support strategizing decisions for successful outcomes and to establish support for positions.

I have had many mentors because I believe that everyone has made a contribution to my life. My most recent mentor is my boss. We share basic beliefs and she allows freedom to reach them in individual ways. Our medicine man has been a great influence as he has facilitated depths of learning that I have searched for my whole life. I do not consider him a mentor because he does not teach, but puts one in touch with truths within. He hands us the keys to unlock our own doors.

S. Rusch

I have not had a mentor, but there are several people whose work and commitment to nursing I greatly admire, e.g., Joyce Clifford.

C. Miller

Mentors have been my mother, a non-nursing supervisor who encouraged me toward a graduate degree in business, and my current supervisor who is the executive director. I am into many "political" problems when a mentor I worked for left the company. I was left to deal with all the people who resented her, and now me.

P. Baumeister

I have had three mentors that have played a very important part in my nursing career at different times. The first mentor was Evelyn Vocelka, RN, the high-school nurse who assisted me in seeing nursing as a possible career choice.

The second mentor was Rita Forelich, RN, MSN. Rita is the owner of the critical-care agency that I have worked for on and off for the past nine years. When I first came to the agency, I was feeling totally burned out and had considered leaving nursing all together. In fact, I had already changed majors. It was Rita's vigorous support of nurses and nursing, her belief that nurses should reap economic benefits from their labor (translated to high salaries), her professionalism, and emphasis on/ support of on-going education and nursing autonomy, that kept me from giving up on my profession. Rita provided a very strong role model for me.

My third mentor was Peggy Chinn, RN, PhD, FAAN, a member of my doctoral committee. When I began working with Peggy, I was again at a critical point. Through Peggy's patient, supportive criticisms of my research and her invaluable suggestions, I was able to grow personally and professionally. I began to see how narrowly I viewed my own nursing career and began to remedy that situation. Peggy provided a very strong role model, and I still depend upon her. I have become more deeply committed to nursing than I ever was before.

There were no negative aspects to having a mentor. I don't think that I would refer to them as "mentors" if the experience wasn't positive.

M. Vrtis

My most significant mentor was a nurse colleague in my fellowship job. She was my main support/teacher/friend in the department (and the only other nurse). She is a leader within the profession. She taught me everything she knows clinically in an unselfish and respectful way. The most important thing she shared was her great sense of idealism and belief in herself and in her practice. She is without apparent self-doubt. If I had an idea, she would say, "Don't apologize! . . . just do it!" The negative aspect of this relationship was that professionally I couldn't visualize us ever being equals. I always carried the sense of being "the student." I decided not to accept a position with her after the fellowship ended, so as to "try my wings" more independently. I still admire her personally and professionally.

In 1982, May, Meleis, and I (1982) explored the opportunities and dilemmas involved in mentoring the fledgling scholar. Those ideas can be extended to other nurse-mentor relationships. We drew six conclusions about mentoring for nursing scholarship, expanded here to include more than the scholar role because the basic ideas are valid for successful nurses.

1. *Roles are developed.* They are created, discovered, and modified over time. They are influenced by significant others, including mentors. They are incorporated into the self and may become relatively enduring aspects of the ever-evolving self.

2. *Roles are interactive in nature.* They exist in the context of others. In order to develop, roles require a chance to be tried and to be challenged. One can fantasize oneself as a clinical specialist, but only practice through interaction with others will make the role a reality.

3. *Education, at any level, prepares one for entry to some aspect of the*

profession. The baccalaureate degree prepares a nurse who is secure and competent to assume general nursing responsibilities. The master's prepares a nurse for entry into specialty practice, and the doctorate provides entry to a research career. Mentorship can enhance the role development of fledglings at all levels.

4. *Women are different than men.* Many of the differences that characterize women are presented as negative by our patriarchical culture, but that is not so. The power-sharing approach often favored by women, as opposed to the power-over approach often favored by men, is often a strength. Women's affiliative needs, achievement orientation, role options, and cognitive preferences need to be taken into account in mentoring. It is generally true that women juggle more roles than men at one time. Women are also newer to the marketplace than men.

5. *Women differ from men in career continuity* (Cole, 1981; Maret, 1983). Women's progress is more likely to be punctuated by role changes (e.g., motherhood), leading to some discontinuity over the career course.

6. *Some of the roles nurses seek, such as researcher, scholar, corporate vice president, and politician, are new for women, and for nurses in particular.* Nurses may experience ambivalence, and the rewards may not be as tangible or as immediate as the nurse is used to in clinical practice.

FUNCTIONS OF MENTORSHIP

Kram (1985) divides the mentoring functions into two broad classes: career and psychosocial. Career functions are direct actions that enhance the chances of success within an organization or discipline. The psychosocial functions are those that create a bond between the mentor and the mentored, and enhance the mentored's sense of professional identity.

The Four Career Functions

Kram mentions four career functions for mentors: sponsorship, leadership, coaching, and protection. Sponsorship is a pragmatic activity directed at helping the person mentored find his or her way in the organization or discipline. It involves speaking up actively about the qualities of the person in meetings, committees, and to persons holding power; it includes introducing the person to the "right people." Sponsorship by only one member of an organization is dangerous, as the person being sponsored may be abandoned if the mentor leaves the organization. Since sponsor acquisition is based upon a genuine appreciation of a person's skills, more than one sponsor can be acquired without violating the mentor relationship.

Sponsorship is a mutually rewarding relationship. Senior persons' reputations are enhanced if they successfully sponsor the next generation's bright organization members. On the flipside, nonsuccessful mentoring of promising new members of the organization may detract from a senior's prestige status.

Another career function of mentoring is creating performance opportunities for a junior, mentored person, including appointments to committees, "blue ribbon" panels, and opportunities for presenting proposals to key persons in the organization. Assignment of the junior person to other parts of the organization that she needs to learn about in order to fulfill her career goals is yet another aspect of mentoring leadership.

Coaching involves teaching strategies and organization politics. It can involve teaching the junior person a new procedure or how to plan a presentation to a committee. It involves sharing the political climate and the senior person's knowledge about what is valued higher up in the organization as well as possible future goals of the organization. This mentoring function is of value no matter how far one progresses in a career. There are always new systems to learn, and a coach can prevent false starts, direct the junior to those persons that will prove helpful, and help steer him or her clear of potentially nonsupportive members of the organization. Coaching also involves feedback about performance; feedback may take the form of telling the junior person what other persons holding power in the organization are saying about her style and knowledge base.

Kram's final career function is protection. The mentor protects the junior person from unjust criticism, jealous rivalry, and from negative exposure to high-risk situations. The mentor may even take the blame for a less-than-successful operation. Protection *can* backfire; it may be valuable for the junior person to face a failure, especially if the issue at hand is not of top-priority nature. Protection can, on the negative side, imply lingering, unstated feelings that the junior person is inept, that the junior person sustains only by merit of the mentor's presence.

Psychosocial Functions

Kram's psychosocial functions of the mentor include role modeling, role clarification, acceptance and confirmation, counseling, and friendship.

Role modeling is essentially a nonverbal behavior in which one performs a role with such precision and completeness that the junior person is able to not only appreciate the role, but emulate it as well. Interviewing can be taught and fledglings can practice it, but there is nothing like watching a master interviewer in action through a one-way mirror; it is electrifying and edifying at the same time.

Hopefully, role modeling does not lead to identification. Junior persons need to develop their own styles based upon the mentor's role incorporated into their own intuition and skills. There is no mentoring if the junior person simply becomes a clone of the senior person. Mentoring should be a dynamic process wherein the junior person develops a strong sense of self-confidence and personal worth. The successful nurse who stated that she did not take a position with her mentor after the fellowship program because she needed to develop her own style was sensitive to this dilemma.

Along with role modeling, the mentor can help in role clarification. In any setting, there is usually a job description. The roles within the job description that are valued and rewarded can be clarified by the mentor. In academia, the role of teacher is truly valued, but fulfilling it alone will seldom lead one to achieve tenure. Scholarly activity, and to a lesser degree community service, are absolutely essential in achieving tenure, no matter what the rhetoric about teaching excellence.

Another aspect of the psychosocial mentoring relationship is the mutually beneficial nature of acceptance and confirmation. For the senior person, the benefits may come later in the career. I guess I have achieved senior-person status because nothing is more pleasing to me than to hear from former students about what they are doing and how much my encouragement meant to them. When I listen to them, I think I must be one of the world's greatest cheer leaders! Acceptance allows the junior persons to rehearse roles. This may literally mean that they will rehearse a new role with the mentor or it may mean that they will be more innovative in their role behaviors because they feel supported by the mentor. This aspect of mentoring requires mutual trust and respect. The junior person must feel secure in that failures are not going to lead to disruption of the relationship.

Mentors counsel. They listen to conflicts, anxieties, and fears that may interfere with productive work. Several of the successful nurses mention that they were the first generation of their family to go to college. Even the most supportive parents, ultimately, cannot understand the challenges and frustrations of the first years on the career ladder. The mentor has been there and can listen and counsel. This function can be crucial for the nurse whose mother is a housewife and cannot help the young career-oriented person balance career, family, and play. I have agonized for mothers who were totally supportive of their daughters, until the daughter decided not to give up her career when the baby arrived. Both mother and daughter disappoint each other. The mother who was deriving satisfaction from the daughter's success now perceives her as a hard career woman who does not care for her child. The daughter, who has basked in the warmth of her mother's approval ever since she can remember, now feels betrayed. A mentor can be helpful here, if asked.

Likewise, a mentor can be helpful when the usually supportive husband suddenly balks at the thought of his wife pursuing graduate study. I have spent lunches and dinners with men who could not understand "what's gotten into her"; who feel she has undergone a personality switch, "she was never like this"; and who perceive the goal as personally threatening. I wish I had the comments of the successful nurses years ago. Graduate education is such a valuable career move for many of them that it might have helped their husbands realize their wives' legitimate goals. In my experience, the question of a graduate degree is not the issue most of the time. In our patriarchal culture, it seems most men do not want their wives pursuing any degree in nursing. The real issue here is change, and whether that change will leave the husband alone or diminished in his wife's eyes.

The last psychosocial function described by Kram is a friendship. Friendship is mutually rewarding; each person has someone to talk with about work and nonwork topics; someone with whom to have lunch. It is, nevertheless, dangerous if this dyad is male-female. Anxieties about gossip and sexual entanglements may limit the friendship function to some extent in cross-sexed mentoring. If the same sexes are involved, the friendships may flourish. Indeed in nursing education, at the graduate level students are sometimes age-peers and colleagues in other settings, so the friendship function can be actualized.

Needs for mentoring vary across career development. The career functions are probably most important when one is beginning a career or making a major shift in career direction. The psychosocial functions can be of value throughout a career.

SELF-ASSESSMENT OF NEED/READINESS FOR A MENTOR

The self-assessment of need for a mentor consists of asking yourself what your goals are. If your goals are to have fun and work just enough to support your hobby, then you probably do not need a mentor. If you want to make quick progress toward a specialization on your career ladder, or toward an administrative position, you could probably benefit from a mentor. If you want to try your skills in several clinical areas in order to decide where you may or may not excel, you may or may not need a mentor. At the same time, you may not attract a mentor because you are unfocused.

Remember that mentor relationships are reciprocal. It is unrealistic to expect someone to recommend you for the right position, or counsel you about the working of the system, if there is a good chance that you will leave or decide to direct your energies to another part of the organization.

If you think a mentor might help you, consider the following:

1. Are you reasonably unsure of the short- and long-term goals of the organization? If your answer is yes and that bothers you, a mentor may be the answer. The sponsorship, coaching, and role-modeling functions may facilitate your career development.

   If your answer is no, a mentor will not be helpful because a mentor is a senior person in the organization and is interesting in furthering the goals of the organization (at least for the time she is there). It is unlikely that you could attract a mentor. You might find someone who could help you clarify your goals.

2. Do you have ideas that could enhance the functioning of the organization? You could use a mentor, especially if you are frustrated because you do not know to whom, or how to communicate them. The sponsorship, exposure/visibility, protection, and role-modeling functions could benefit you.

3. If your clinical/academic skills are growing, but you need a broader audience with whom to share them, you are a great candidate for mentoring. You need exposure and visibility, as well as the acceptance/confirmation and counseling functions.

4. Are peers and supervisors saying, "You have great ideas, if you could just learn to present them in a way that is constructive." You may benefit from a mentor or you may need psychotherapy or counseling.

If the problem is that you simply do not know how to market or present ideas, a mentor will suffice. If you have an underlying insecurity that manifests in putting others down, or in being overly aggressive or defensive, a mentor will not help. Remember, a mentor is part of the system, and so cannot afford to sponsor someone who has already been labeled a "troublemaker" or "crazy." Your chances of attracting a mentor are further diminished if your academic credentials and clinical/administrative skills are not very good.

5. Are you always in trouble? This may mean that you are not accomplished in certain required skills and knowledges. A friend or a supervisor at evaluation time could probably tell you this. There is a possibility that you could use a mentor to protect you, but if you are already perceived as disruptive to the goals of the system, you probably will not find one. Remember, mentoring is not a rescue operation. If you decide that you really got carried away, it may be better to go to another setting and start again, or make it clear to colleagues and superiors that you are changing. As one of the successful nurses pointed out, to be in trouble for the right reason is a fine thing; however, it is often hard to determine if this is the case. We do tend to be very convinced of our own righteousness.

6. Are you lonely at work? A mentor is not the answer. Friendship is the least-often fulfilled mentoring function because of the social complications inherent in being friends with persons who may be on different rungs of the hierarchical ladder. Friendship is a by-product of mentoring, not the motivation for it.

7. Are you underachieving in your eyes and in the eyes of your colleagues, in spite of expert skills and knowledge? You may desperately need a mentor. If you are unsophisticated in system politics, there may be an enemy blocking your road to visibility and important assignments. A mentor would assess this situation fairly rapidly and use the sponsorship, exposure/visibility, coaching, protection, role-modeling, and acceptance/confirmation roles to get you over this impasse.

8. Do you want to change the direction of your career? A mentor, or several mentors, may be called for. One mentor may be good at assessing the functional/transferable skills you have to take to another career. Another mentor may facilitate your departure from

your current track without alienating other people. For a powerful person to say, "Jane was using about 50% percent of her potential as a manager; I really encourage her to pursue the doctorate," can go a long way in alleviating the feeling of abandonment in former colleagues. If you couple this with a series of I-statements about your frustration with your current status (not a series of statements about how dreadful "they" are and "things" are) and proactive goals for your future, you can leave former colleagues with a sense of their worth and with a feeling of happiness for your new career choice. Do remember, there are those people in the world who never rejoice in anything but bad news, those who suffer from "terminal" jealousy, and those who need to think that you were miserably unhappy because they are. Most people, however, will respond positively to honest changes for self-improvement. Even if you were unhappy, that is a learning and there is no need to denigrate people who find fulfillment where you could not. No system is perfect; every system must have something to offer someone or it would cease to exist.

LOOSE ENDS

Mentoring is a complex interpersonal, emotional relationship. Mentors are senior persons in an organization; they are not there to foment rebellion or to create chaos. Indeed, if you sensed that from a would-be "mentor," run; they may plan to use you to do their dirty work. A mentor is a pillar of the organization and can teach you how the organization works and how you can prosper within it. If you are a revolutionary or someone who wants to disrupt the organization, would-be mentors will avoid you. Remember, their success in sponsoring the organization's or discipline's next generation of leaders is their reward for mentoring.

Another loose end has to do with protection and independence (May, Meleis, & Winstead-Fry, 1982). Nursing is a young profession. We are not always sure of our footing, especially at the corporate level and in scholarly roles. Risk taking is feared by some women. A mentor, even with the best of intentions, may overprotect. This will squash creativity and independence, giving way to mentor "cloning."

The other loose end in mentoring is exploitation. I have heard as many stories about the mentor being exploited as I have heard about the junior person being exploited. In some service settings, persons with baccalaureate, and even higher degrees, are so rare that they cluster together, often forming rather desperate relationships. Sometimes these are mistaken for mentoring relationships. However, the junior person is using the senior person to learn enough to oust her. Real mentoring is based on mutual respect and trust. If you feel that you are giving more than you are receiving, you are not in a mentorship relationship. On the other hand, I do know of a few senior people who take the research ideas of bright junior faculty/staff. In all, nothing is perfect. Do not give unconditional trust without some indication that it is returned. Also beware of the new, untried mentor. One of the great challenges to the mentor is to encourage persons who are/may be better than you. I can remember one of the truly great mentors in my life who flatly said that she was glad she was 30 years older than I because she would hate to compete with me. The overly competitive mentor creates disaster! The junior person will either become her pawn or the scapegoat for problems caused by mentor's own overcompetitiveness.

The last loose end is to beware the protégé role. It is likely that sometimes hero/heroine worship is at play when a mentoring relationship develops, especially when the relationship is initiated by the junior person. If the junior person is forever performing menial tasks, she is not being sponsored—she is being used, not mentored. Traditional women are used to pleasing, and to please a person of high status may feel right, but it is not mentoring. A mentor should push a junior person toward challenges, increase a junior person's visibility, and become excited by the junior person's achievements.

9

Assertiveness

I learned to be more assertive during my years as a clinical nurse specialist. I don't think I ever learned to be assertive very well. A lot has to do with other people's perceptions and sometimes I thought I was really being effective, but the person I was dealing with was offended or insulted or whatever. I have never studied assertiveness training. I'm still really old fashioned about it. I was raised to be kind to other people and they would in turn be kind to me. Can you imagine the reality shock that hit this kid as a new staff nurse at Boston University Medical Center at the tender age of 21!

I am assertive and I have taken courses. I teach it, practice it, model it, and use it in collaboration and negotiation. I believe that you won't know if you don't ask. Know what you want and let others know and attempt to get it. Simultaneously, respect others' rights to want something different.

Assertiveness is very important in being a nurse. I developed the skill during my first few years as a new graduate. I've always been a self-confident person which made it easy to then become assertive once I was confident with my nursing skills and knowledge.

D. Boyle

I have read about assertiveness and understand the concept. I don't consider myself assertive enough for an administrative position. I don't like making decisions for other people. I have tried to be more assertive in my personal life, and found I seem to hurt people; so I don't try to be assertive any more. At work, my attitude is everyone has to work together to get the job done and I must be assertive enough to get the job done. I would never go to an assertiveness-training workshop because I know I would hate it and I have decided that I'm just fine the way I am.

J. Sheehy

Some might say in my early career I was more aggressive than assertive. That is why I actively sought help in my ability to communicate. Now I tend to interact in a much gentler and still effective fashion. Yes, I would say I am very assertive.

M. Gorman

I taught assertiveness training. I have mixed feelings about it. Assertiveness training is consonant with an individual having a problem, rather than society having a problem, and thus may be seen as another way of keeping oppressed groups down. Besides, who gets to decide what's assertive and what's aggressive?

My unanswered question is why do so many similar types of individuals, for example women, have problems with assertiveness? This assumes that the problem belongs to women and ignores the context.

In my experience, when you choose to stick your neck out, you can expect to have it chopped off now and then. If you choose not to stick your neck out, you lose opportunities. Also, you have to live with yourself. Sometimes not taking a chance is harder than sticking your neck out in the first place.

K. Allman

I have taught assertiveness to staff nurses and have learned to apply the concepts to my own life. The concepts have become more natural to me. Being married to a chauvinistic male indeed has tested my assertiveness to the limit, and required me to learn how to deal with aggressive behavior.

P. Iyer

. . . I've never taken assertiveness training. I think that one needs to be honest and respectful, and deal with things as they happen, with persistence, if the situation is not remedied. I rather take a tai-chi stance, that is, moving with the force rather than directly confronting it with force. Using positives rather than negatives in one's approach, as well as referring to "I" rather than "you" in a discussion, goes a long way in improving communication.

D. Calvani

I tend to be rather shy, but know I am very knowledgeable in my field of ophthalmic nursing and am able to express an opinion with confidence. However, this type of assertiveness is construed as being abrasive when there is a dispute and someone's lack of knowledge is shown up. If there is something that needs to be done, I will certainly take the lead in getting it done, and then stick to the cause until the challenge is completed.

H. Boyd-Monk

To accomplish anything today in such a frantic world, one must be assertive enough to stay in the mainstream. It is too easy to be left at the wayside waiting for the right opportunity to come along. If I know something or want to do something, I speak up. It may be that I may not get exactly what I am asking for, but I have let myself be heard. If my patients had needs to be met, I had to be assertive enough to follow through. Why not the same for myself? With all my formal education, and the continuing-education offerings I have attended, yes, I have had some assertiveness training.

J. Sage

I utilize assertive behaviors consistently. I am aware of others' needs in the process and am usually able to assertively achieve my goals without preventing others from doing the same in the process. I am capable of being very aggressive, losing all sensitivity to others in those moments when I feel most angry or threatened. I usually end up regretting this steamroller behavior of mine, and go about trying to clean up after my storm.

I have not taken assertiveness training. I have read many articles and some books on the topic.

Being assertive is a positive experience for me in that I express my needs, request support for them, and usually get a positive response even if negotiation is required. When I am overtly aggressive and inattentive to those around me, I may get my needs met, but usually suffer some cost in other ways; such as loss of communication with others, guilt from acting in an uncaring manner, loss of companionship, etc.

S. L. McAllister

My assertiveness training came from the feminist movement in the early 1970s. Reading in sexual awareness and an increasing awareness of gender biases in society, in my marriage, and in nursing. My growth in this area came with my struggle to help my women patients with their struggles with these issues.

M. Sprik

I haven't studied assertiveness training, but I think I am fairly assertive by nature. I don't view this as having had a major effect on my career development thus far. I think it will be important in employment situations once I complete my doctoral studies.

I have had assertiveness training. It was and is good for me. As long as I draw the line and never cross over to aggressiveness. This is where I feel that many go wrong, and I also used to make that mistake.

Assertiveness! I wish I had it! I keep promising myself to take a course someday. Little by little, time and experience are bestowing it upon me.

G. Wall

I think I consider myself mildly assertive. I am comfortable being assertive for what I believe in . . . I do create opportunities to be assertive. I am not comfortable yet with open conflict; so the opportunities I create are in scholarly forums, structured, I guess, versus spontaneous. I think more of my assertiveness as a tool for survival, rather than a tool for advancement. I do not think my assertiveness has played a major role in my career success. I have not studied assertiveness training.

G. Mitchel

My thesis was on assertiveness. At that time, I studied it in depth. I believe I am primarily assertive. Sometimes, I slip into passivity. I am quite intent on protecting the rights of myself and others. I have never been sorry that I appreciate being in trouble for the right reason.

I have had to use assertiveness to some extent to achieve my goals, but it has been a struggle for me to be assertive each time it was required. So I don't see it as being a large part of my career development, although I know it has been.

R. Brown

If by assertiveness you mean clear and confident expression of needs, beliefs, [and] goals, then I think that assertiveness has been critical in my ability to achieve my goals. Although I have not studied assertiveness training, I think that this is a skill that I have been developing for some time with more confidence in some areas than in others. Assertiveness was an important component of my education and practice as a nurse practitioner. To make an impact in an interdisciplinary, often physician-dominated setting, you had to value your nursing perspective and make sure it was heard. As I gain more experience and confidence in my skills as a nurse scientist, I expect that my comfort with assertiveness will grow in this domain as well.

These successful nurses' comments define the term assertiveness skills: the ability to pursue a goal to completion with respect for one's self and for others. Whether or not these nurses had formal assertiveness training, they have learned the behaviors that lead to effective assertiveness.

Assertiveness, rather than aggression, is the survival skill for anyone who is committed to achieving anything. Assertiveness is planned, and begins with the self: One sets limits and is honest and clear about one's goals. To randomly attack family or colleagues who we may perceive as performing some activity unsatisfactorily, when that activity has been ill-defined does not constitute "assertiveness," but rather aggression, and plain bad manners.

We all behave poorly at times—"overly aggressive" to use S. L. McAllister's words—and sometimes realize our behavior only when we've realized how unclear we were about our goals. For example, we can imagine wanting to bomb a nursing unit (after removing all of the patients, of course) because the nursing staff mismanaged the collection of some data. In the course of being "overly aggressive" we may come to realize that we may well have been ambivalent about the research project. Once we cool off, we can re-examine the pros and cons of the project; we may come to realize that we had set up the data collection in such a way that it was bound to fail, had we not been present at a couple of critical junctures. Of course, our schedules could not ensure our presence at those times, so the project floundered. Once our goals are respectfully and assertively clarified, we can return to the staff involved and work out a far better data-collection method.

Probably the best way to decide if your goals are clear is to answer the question, "Can I state the goal in one or two simple sentences with action verbs?" This is the same basic idea that was discussed in goal setting for career planning. If you cannot clearly state the goal to yourself, it is quite likely that you cannot state it intelligibly to others.

A classic exercise in behavioral training in assertiveness involves practice in not buying something from a door-to-door sales representative. The key to successful completion of this exercise is a clear commitment to yourself that you are not going to buy what the salesperson is offering. Once that commitment is clear, the various techniques of assertiveness training are learned without the perception of gimmickry. You begin to see the techniques as legitimate tools to accomplish your goal of not purchasing the product.

Another aspect of the self in assertiveness has to do with voice. If you sound childlike, or are so soft-voiced that people cannot hear you, you need to correct this before you can become assertive. Borisoff's (1985) work on women's voices is illustrative of these unique issues for women. Women are, and have been socialized to believe that a pleasing feminine voice is soft and sweet. An effective voice is firm and well modulated (not shouting and angry—that signifies aggression). In business situations, softly phrased sentences, no matter how pertinent, are not heard.

When a soft voice emanates from a small body, the potential for not being heard becomes great. I call this the "Barbie doll" problem. The model for effective leaders is male. Even within the male group, leaders are typically six feet tall, fairly muscular, and have "strong" voices. If you look over photographs of the presidents of Fortune-500 corporations, you will find few men who do not fulfill this stereotype. A woman who looks like a Barbie doll and has a soft voice is at a disadvantage. There are various techniques to overcome this, such as wearing hats that increase the illusion of height. However, these all take too much time for practicality, and cost money. Also, these techniques do not address the issue of assertiveness.

Your voice is the easiest thing to change to combat the "Barbie doll" problem. You can learn to speak distinctly, in a medium-pitch range, and with conviction. All it takes is practice in front of the mirror, and then in public. One of the most effective nurse administrators I know is about five-foot three and weighs probably 100 pounds. She has a clear, concise, and well-modulated verbal style. I have enjoyed asking males and females to describe her to me. Invariably, something such as, "Oh, she is about five-feet seven . . . ," is included in their descriptions. This woman's self-confident skills and assertive presence add four inches to people's perceptions of her height.

A proper understanding of assertiveness skills requires from the start, that one's goals are clear and that one's skills are likewise well developed. Several of these successful nurses comment that they had to develop sound clinical judgment before being assertive for self or client. It is almost impossible for nurses to accomplish their goal if they are not respected as experts in clinical practice.

Assertiveness also involves other factors. Body language is important. If you blush, become silent, shy away, or cannot maintain direct eye contact, no matter how clearly you articulate your ideas, you will create less of an impact. Assessment of your body language is difficult; our body language is so much a part of who we are that we are seldom aware of it. The two easiest behaviors to identify are lack of eye contact and becoming silent. If you get tongue-tied and begin to study the floor when you find yourself in an anxious situation, you need to practice asserting yourself. A mentor can be very helpful here, as can friends and colleagues. You might practice speaking up and being heard with these persons. You can set a goal of looking everyone straight in the eye, regardless of situation, until this behavior begins to feel natural.

What you have to say also contributes to your assertiveness. If you know little about a subject, it is better not to assert an opinion. If you cannot accept the consequences of a statement/action at the moment, do not do it.

Respecting others' rights and needs is a part of assertiveness. To do otherwise constitutes aggression. Assertiveness does not mean forcing your choices upon the other person; they have a right to choose their own behaviors and responses to your behavior. Choice for all involved is a goal of assertiveness. Denying your needs openly, but being manipulative backhandedly, likewise does not constitute assertiveness, even if you are successful in getting what you want. All of us have experienced sitting at a table where everyone voices an opinion on some issue and votes for some active decision, only to have the decision rescinded because some participant denied or did not assert their honest opinion, but manipulated the group with side issues of little consequence. For example, I was once in a group where a powerful nurse educator sat mutely through meetings, but always voted with the majority. After the meeting, she would call members and invite them to "rethink" the decision. Her actions often led to confusion and quarreling within the group. Group members present become justifiably angry, not only for the manipulation, but for the waste of time spent at the meeting. Being unprepared for a meeting is bad, but being unassertive about your true feelings or ideas probably wastes more meeting time than any other single issue.

SELF-ASSESSMENT

1. Self Factors:

   a. Do I know what my goals are in this situation?

   b. Can I express my goals clearly in a brief sentence or two?

   c. Do I sound firm and strong when I speak about my goals?

   d. Do I respect the values and goals of the people I am trying to influence?

   e. Can I accept negative consequences of my assertions?

   f. Am I relaxed, well prepared, and can I project my enthusiasm about this project or idea?

2. Social Factors:

   a. Is this the right time for me to make this assertion?

   b. Is this the right place for me to do this?

   c. Am I prepared to deal with being successful?

   d. Can I implement this goal with my current resources?

   e. Do I have enough support for this project to have a reasonable chance for success?

   f. Can I deal with the social/organizational consequences of not getting my request?

If your answer to all of these questions is yes, you are truly in a rare and enviable position. Usually, one should answer yes to the self factors before asserting some goal in a business setting. If there are too many no's in the social-factor assessment, rethink whether the time to ask for something is appropriate. Regardless of the career stage that you are in, developing a reputation as someone who lets colleagues, clients, or the organization down is to be avoided.

Assertive Rights

Smith (1975), in his best-seller, *When I Say No, I Feel Guilty*, proposes a Bill of Assertive Rights. These are worth reviewing because they summarize neatly what one hopes to achieve through assertiveness.

1. You have the right to judge your own behavior, thoughts and emotions, and to take responsibility for their initiation and consequences to yourself.

2. You have the right to offer no excuses for justifying your behavior.

3. You have the right to judge if you are responsible for finding solutions to other people's problems.

4. You have the right to change your mind.

5. You have the right to make mistakes and to be responsible for them.

6. You have the right to say, "I don't know."

7. You have the right to be independent of the goodwill of others before coping with them.

8. You have the right to be illogical in making decisions.

9. You have the right to say, "I don't understand."

10. You have the right to say, "I don't care."

11. You have the right to say no, without feeling guilty.

This Bill of Assertive Rights can also serve as an assessment tool to determine how well you are doing in setting respectful and realistic boundaries for yourself in regard to the demands of others. They capture concisely the dimensions of responsibility and right. The integration of these two dimensions of assertiveness is what separates assertiveness from aggression, on one hand, and wimpiness, on the other. Both wimpiness and aggression are counter-productive to developing a career of which you and others can be proud.

References

Baer, E. (1982). *The conflictive social ideology of American nursing: 1893, a microcosm.* Unpublished doctoral dissertation, New York University.

Barrett, E. M. (1989). Power as knowing participation in change. In J. Riehl-Sisca (Ed.), *Conceptual models for nursing practice* (3rd ed.). Norwalk, CT: Appleton & Lange.

Belenky, M. F., Clinchy, B., Goldberger, N. R., & Tarule, J. M. (1986). *Women's ways of knowing.* New York: Basic Books.

Bolen, J. S. (1984). *Goddesses in everywomen.* New York: Harper & Row.

Bolles, R. N. (1981). *The three boxes of life.* Berkeley, CA: Ten Speed Press.

Bolles, R. N. (1985). *What color is your parachute?* Berkeley, CA: Ten Speed Press.

Bolles, R. N., & Zenoff, V. B. (1977). *The quick job hunters map.* Berkeley, CA: Ten Speed Press.

Borisoff, D., & Berrill, L. (1985). *The power to communicate.* Prospect Heights, IL: Waveland Press.

Boszormenyi-Nagy, I., & Spark, G. M. (1973). *Invisible loyalties.* New York: Harper & Row.

Bowen, M. (1978). *Family theory in clinical practice.* New York: Jason Aronson.

Brooks, L. (1984). Counseling special groups: Women and ethnic minorities. In D. Brown, L. Brooks, & Associates (Eds.), *Career choice and development.* San Francisco: Jossey-Bass.

Brooten, D., Kumar, S., Brown, L., Butts, P., Finkler, S., Bakewell-Sachs,

P., Gibbons, A., & Delivoria-Papadoponlus, M. (1986). A randomized clinical trial of early hospital discharge and home follow-up of very-low-birth weight infants. *New England Journal of Medicine, 315,* 934–939.

Connell, M. T. (1983). Feminine consciousness and the nature of nursing practice. *Topics in Clinical Nursing, 5,* 1–10.

Erikson, E. (1968). *Identity: Youth and crisis.* New York: W. W. Norton.

Erikson, E., Erikson, J. M., & Kivnick, H. Q. (1986). *Vital involvement in old age.* New York: W. W. Norton.

Fagin, C. (1986). Opening the door on nursing's cost advantage. *Nursing and Health Care, 7,* 356–358.

Fitzgerald, L. F., & Crites, J. O. (1980). Toward a career psychology of women: What do we know? What do we need to know? *Journal of Counseling Psychology, 27,* 44–62.

Frankl, V. (1958). *Man's search for meaning.* Boston: Beacon Press.

Gilligan, C. (1982). *In a different voice.* Cambridge, MA: Harvard University Press.

Guerin, P. J., & Pendagast, E. G. (1976). Evaluation of family system and genogram. In P. J. Guerin, Jr. (Ed.), *Family therapy: Theory and practice.* New York: Gardner Press.

Hennig, M., & Jardim, A. (1977). *The managerial woman.* New York: Pocket Books.

Herrmann, N. (1988). *The creative brain.* Lake Lurie, NC: Brain Books.

Miller, S. M., & Winstead-Fry, P. (1982). *Family systems theory in nursing practice.* Reston, VA: Reston Publishing.

Jennings, D. (1987). *Self-made women.* Dallas: Taylor Publishing.

Josefwitz, N. (1980). *Paths to power.* Reading, MA: Addison-Wesley.

Jung, G. C. (1973). *Synchronicity* (R. F. C. Hull, Trans., Bollingen Series). Princeton: Princeton University Press.

Keyes, R. (1985). *Chancing it.* Boston: Little Brown.

Knowles, E. S. (1976). Search for motivation in risk-taking and gambling. In W. Eadington (Ed.), *Gambling and society.* Springfield, IL: Charles C. Thomas.

Kohlberg, L. (1984). *The psychology of moral development.* New York: Harper & Row.

Kram, K. E. (1985). *Mentoring at work.* Glenview, IL: Scott, Foresman and Co.

Levinson, D. J. (1978). *The seasons of a man's life*. New York: Alfred A. Knopf.

Loughary, J., & Ripley, T. (1977). *Life planning training program: Self-empowerment*. Unpublished manuscript. Eugene, OR: University of Oregon.

Mason, D. J., & Talbott, S. W. (1985). *Political action handbook for nurses*. Menlo Park, CA: Addison-Wesley.

May, K., Meleis, A., & Winstead-Fry, P. (1982). Mentorship for scholarliness: Opportunities and dilemmas. *Nursing Outlook*, 30(1), 22–28.

McClure, M., Poulin, M., Sovie, M., & Wandelt, M. (1983). *Magnet hospitals*. Kansas City: American Nurses' Association.

Miller, S., & Winstead-Fry, P. (1982). Family systems theory in nursing practice. Reston, VA: Reston Publishing.

Moran, P. (1983). *Invest in yourself: A women's guide to starting her own business*. Garden City, NY: Dolphin.

Neugarten, B. L. (1969). Continuities and discontinuities of psychological issues into adult life. *Human Development, 12*, 121–130.

Piaget, J. (1952). *The language and thought of the child*. London: Routledge & Kegan Paul.

Punch, L. (1983). Nursing 'foremen' hold key to productivity under DRG system. *Modern Healthcare, 3*(7), 152–154.

Rose, S. (1986). *Career guide for women scholars*. New York: Springer.

Rossi, A. (1980). Aging and parenting in the middle years. In P. Baltes & O. Brim Jr. (Eds.), *Life span development and behavior: Vol. 3*. New York: Academic Press.

Sher, B. (1979). *Wishcraft: How to get what you really want*. New York: Ballantine Books.

Siegelman, E. Y. (1983). *Personal risk*. New York: Harper & Row.

Smith, M. (1975). *When I say no, I feel guilty*. New York: Bantam Books.

Van Maanen, J., & Schein, E. H. (1977). Career development. In J. Richard Hackman and J. Lloyd Suttle (Eds.), *Improving life at work*. Santa Monica, CA: Goodyear.

Vogel, G., & Doleysh, N. (1988). *Entrepreneuring: A nurse's guide to starting a business*. New York: National League for Nursing.

Appendix

QUESTIONNAIRE FOR PARTICIPATING NURSES

Please read the questions and think about them. Place your ideas and responses on the lined, colored paper provided. Please feel free to add more paper. A stamped, self-addressed envelope is included for your convenience.

Please check your choice:

_____ You may identify me by name and state (e.g., S. Smith of Oregon).

_____ Please do not identify me by name.

1. My age is _____ .

2. My sex is _____ .

3. I work in an urban, suburban, or rural location (circle one).

4. I have been a nurse for _____ years.

5. I have been in my current position for _____ years.

6. My first degree in nursing was _____ .

7. The highest degree I hold in nursing is _____ .

8. The highest degree I hold in another discipline is _____ .

9. What attracted you to the nursing profession?

10. The literature on career development distinguishes a career from a job in that a career involves choice, meaningful responsibility, personal rewards, and a degree of economic security. I wonder, did you always view nursing as a career or did you, at some point, see it as a job (regular schedule with a paycheck)?

    If you perceived nursing as a job, what led to perceiving it as a career?

    If you always perceived nursing as a career, how did you come to this awareness? Some people have a mentor; others parental guidance; sometimes there is a critical incident, such as a divorce; sometimes there are multiple factors. How was it for you?

11. Have you done career planning or career mapping?

    If yes, by what method?

    If no, do you have an intuitive sense of how you will make progress?

    Some of you may have both an intuitive sense and a plan. Regardless of your approach, please discuss how you achieved your current goal(s) and where you want to be in five years.

12. Was (is) risk taking a skill you developed to achieve your goals? I would appreciate a vignette(s) about risks taken; ideas you have on how to minimize dangerous risks and what you consider reasonable risks.

13. Do you have a style of making decisions? Most of the career planning/ management literature favors a rational–logical approach to decision making. What is your experience with decision making? Are you intuitive as well as rational? Do you have a formula or set of rules that guide your decision-making processes? What do you consider the best decision you have made to date about your career (or about how to balance career and personal life)?

14. To what extent has formal education been a tool for career advancement? To what extent has informal/continuing education been a tool for career advancement?

15. How have you managed "the system" to your advantage? Please write a bit about the system in which you work and about the nursing system with which you interact.

16. What personal strengths do you have that make you successful? Did you develop these strengths through effort or were they a natural part of your personality? What weaknesses or limitations do you grapple with?

17. I would like to know a bit about your family, how you grew up, and significant choices in your life that influenced your career path. For example, I am sure that the fact that I am the first-born girl in a fairly traditional family had a great deal to do with my becoming a nurse.

18. Have you had a mentor(s)? How has the mentor facilitated your career? Did you experience any negative aspects of having a mentor?

19. To what extent have you used assertiveness to achieve your goals? Have you studied assertiveness training? What is your experience with being assertive?

THANK YOU